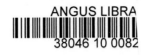

YOGA for Cancer

|| Esoteric, Yogic & Dietary Remedies ||

YOGA for Cancer

|| Esoteric, Yogic & Dietary Remedies ||

BIJOYLAXMI HOTA

Recipes by
Carissa Leventis-Cox

Rupa & Co

Text Copyright © Bijoylaxmi Hota 2009
Design Copyright © Rupa & Co. 2009

First Published 2009
Second Impression 2010

Published by
Rupa Publications India Pvt. Ltd.
7/16, Ansari Road, Daryaganj
New Delhi 110 002

Sales Centres:

Allahabad Bengaluru Chandigarh Chennai
Hyderabad Jaipur Kathmandu
Kolkata Mumbai

Designed and illustrated by
Ishtihaar

Printed in India by
Nutech Photolithographers
B-240, Okhla Industrial Area, Phase-I,
New Delhi 110 020, India

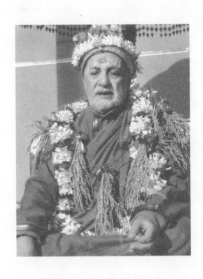

With the blessings
of my Guru and Guide

Paramhamsa Swami Satyananda Saraswati

Contents

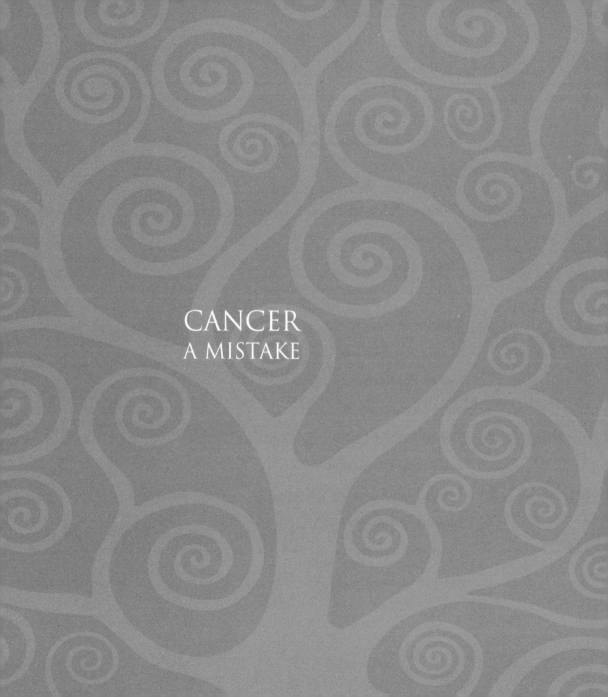

CANCER
A MISTAKE

Cancer – A Mistake

We exist because nature has made survivors of us all, from that miniscule microbe to the complex rational homo sapiens. Modern science has recently commenced looking into the mysterious workings of the living body. As for the mind boggling complexities of the human body, the voyage has only just begun. For long, western science had pooh-poohed the 'miracles' of eastern health systems, dismissing them as tricks and con jobs. Gradually though, there has been an attempt to understand the learning behind these miracles. Yoga is a vast and ancient body of knowledge, a collection of wisdom on how the human body, mind and psyche form an unbroken whole. Hence, the 'miracles' – Yogis have walked on fire and on water, stayed without oxygen or gone without food for months. The famous British travel writer Paul Brunton along with the Indian Nobel Laureate Jagdish Chandra Bose, witnessed how Trailangya Swami drank sulphuric acid followed by potassium cyanide without coming to any harm. In a mortuary in Los Angeles, Swami Yoganand's body showed no signs of decay even twenty days after his death.

Yoga believes that the cause, the manifestation and the cure all lie within the individual. In other words, the prevention and the cure of an ailment are within the grasp of the individual. You can diagnose and treat yourself. If that is not empowerment, then what is? Yoga taps into the limitless reserves of the vital energy that nature has equipped us with. Remember, we are all survivors! Yoga activates this dormant power to allow us to heal ourselves. In yoga, you take the responsibility of your wellbeing. You do not surrender yourself to an impersonal, mass produced system of medicine and pharmacopeia that strips you of your individuality and reduces you to an entry in the hospital records. With yoga, you assume command of your life, your health and your happiness! You can see that the ancient knowledge of yoga is extremely modern. By making us conscious of that healing power residing in us, yoga empowers us to take on any ailment, physical or mental, and even the most debilitating ailment known to man – cancer.

Modern medicine in its fight against cancer turns the patient into a helpless and passive recipient of therapy. The allopathic pharmacopeia is a double-edged sword. The highly potent drugs have such toxic side-effects that they leave the patient feeling more ill than before. As yoga is a drugless therapy, the possibility of deleterious side-effects do not arise. Yoga relies not on external and artificially created inputs, but, on the energy and the will of the patient. All it requires is a sincere adherence to yoga for healing the body. But, by yoga I do not mean only *asanas* and *pranayamas*. Besides these there are many other yogic practices which are explained in this book, *Yoga for Cancer*.

In my years of practice, I have seen the effectiveness of yogic treatment on many of my patients. A few of them had the following to say:

'I was put onto chemotherapy after the removal of a malignant tumor which had affected my breast and glands. I practiced yoga under the guidance of Mrs Bijoylaxmi Hota because of which I did not suffer the side effects of chemotherapy such as hair and energy loss. My immunity which became extremely low went up to measure over 95 per cent in about six months.'

Edith Pfiester
Switzerland

Yoga's effect on abnormal tissue growth is phenomenal. A case worth mentioning here is that of Dr Vandana's. In her own words:

'I underwent a major surgery at the John's Hopkins Hospital in Baltimore to have a very large rapidly growing tumor removed. Since then, I was taking medication as a preventive. Three months later, when I went for a check-up, a larger tumor was found. I came to Delhi and learnt yoga under Mrs Hota. In one month's time, the tumor disappeared. My surgeon in Baltimore said the disappearance of the tumor was nothing short of a miracle. If he did not have the earlier film to compare it with, he would not have believed such a thing was possible.'

Dr Vandana Chandra
Baltimore, US

Right diet is crucial in enhancing the potency of yogic treatment. An appropriate diet can sometimes act as the most important weapon in arresting and reversing the growth of cancer, as I found in the case of a relative. This girl was diagnosed with a large uterine tumor. She was advised immediate surgery. She, however, put her faith in yoga and came to me for help. As she could not perform most of the recommended *asanas* due to severe lower back pain, I taught her a few very simple ones and concentrated more on her diet. Within a month, the tumor had been reduced to half!

The above mentioned cases are not flukes, rather they represent the large number of cancer patients who have found health and hope through the revitalising and life enhancing powers of yoga. You too can take charge of restoring your wellbeing! But before taking up any of these practices take the consent of the doctor treating you as she or he knows your condition better.

CHAPTER I

PRANA AND PRANAYAMA

Prana and *Pranayama*

What is the difference between us and the dust particles? Aren't we both composed of the same metals and chemicals and aren't we both the same congealed energy? What actually sets us apart, is the presence of the life current in our body that yoga calls *prana*. It is this *prana* that animates the inanimate. As long as it remains in the body, the individual lives, breathes and eats and when it leaves, death ensues.

Prana is not an imaginary new substance. Ancient cultures around the world have been aware of its presence since antiquity. They have called it by various names such as *Qui*, *Chi* and *Manna*. Many healing methods such as acupressure, acupuncture, reiki and pranic healing have been developed on the basis of this energy. Now scientists, too, have acknowledged the existence of this energy.

In 1935, a professor of neuro-anatomy at the Yale University, USA, discovered that an energy field enveloped all animate objects and he called it the Electro Dynamic Field. A few years later, Mr Kirlian invented the now famous Kirlian camera that could capture *prana* in all its hues and forms. Subsequently, Dr Hiroshi Motoyama tracked down its movement in the human body with a scientific instrument. Thereafter, Dr Nagahama at Chiba Medical School in Japan, measured the velocity of *prana* and proved that it was not electric energy produced by the nerve, as suspected by many, because the time *prana* took to pass any distance was much slower than the nerve conduction. The energy was not found to be magnetic either. Finally, scientists accepted it and called it the bio-plasmic energy.

The strength of *prana* in a human body determines the level of energy and state of health of that person. It is believed that more the *prana*, the more energetic one feels and the healthier one remains. It is a misconception that muscles determine our energy levels. If that was the case, the continuous activities of small children, with hardly any bulky muscles, would be a surprise!

Most people are born with an abundant supply of *prana,* but it does not remain constant and gets depleted for various reasons. Both Indian yogis as well as Russian scientists have observed that one needs a continuous replenishment of this vital force to remain in good health. Yoga regards *prana* as the most powerful healing energy, which we absorb from the atmosphere through our natural breathing process. But how much of it do we actually receive depends on the air surrounding us. In stuffy city rooms, there is never

enough *prana* for perfect health. Scientific instruments have measured the maximum density of this energy in the mountains. Next come sea shores and riverbanks. Sometimes, concerned physicians advice their patients a 'change of place', and those who go to the above mentioned places seem to benefit the most. In the past, before TB drugs were discovered, many TB patients, who went to live in the hills recovered completely.

Even though there is not much *prana* in the cities, the available amount can be amplified through yoga. A set of specific breathing exercises called *pranayama* absorb the maximum amount of *prana* from the atmosphere. Though, now being used for health reasons, the original purpose of *pranayama* was different. They were devised to create a yogic fire in the body to heat and awaken the *kundalini* – the dormant serpent power present near the tailbone of every human being.

Kundalini is no myth. From time to time, evolved souls have been born with an awakened *kundalini*, and have exhibited unimaginable power. Meerabai, the most significant figures of Indian *bhakti* tradition is a prime example. She was born into a royal Rajput family of Mewar and early in her childhood itself, she had announced to her family that she would marry Lord Krishna and saw the lord everywhere and in everything. Nobody and nothing else existed for her. When it was time for her to marry, she was wedded to the prince of Chhitorgarh, but her behaviour did not change. She lived in her own world, dancing and singing the praise of Lord Krishna. Embarrassed by her behaviour and suspecting her to be having an affair with another man, her in-laws decided to kill her. One day, they sent Meera a basket with a cobra inside and a message that the basket contained a garland of flowers. She opened the basket and was surprised to find a lovely idol of Lord Krishna with a garland of flowers. Then, they sent her a cup of poison with the message that it was nectar. Meera offered it to her Lord Krishna and drank it as His blessing and it actually turned into nectar! Not the ones to give up, they sent her a bed of nails, but when she reposed on it, it transformed into a bed of roses.

In this way, all their attempts to end Meera's life failed. She lived on for many more years and when the time came for her to leave this world, she is said to have entered the sanctum sanctorum of a temple and locked herself in. After sometime, when the door was broken open, there was nobody inside. It is believed that, Meerabai transformed herself into pure energy and merged with the all-pervading cosmic energy.

Yogic texts indicate that, nothing is impossible for a person with an awakened *kundalini*, and the yogis who were aware of it devised various means to achieve that. One of the methods was *pranayama*. Barring a few of them which have a cooling effect on the body, most *pranayamas* generate heat. However, if the heat becomes too strong, the mucus membrane begins to dry up inside the body, which can prove to be detrimental to one's health.

Yogis, who aim for such intense heat for the great awakening, take a special diet and practice *kriyas* to protect themselves. But for the rest of us, it is better not to do *pranayama* for more than half an hour daily.

Cancer, considered a cold disease by yoga responds well to the heat producing *pranyamas* such as *bhastrika* and *suryabheda*. Ideally, *pranayams* should be practiced during sunrise or sunset when the sky has a red tinge, as at this time the *prana* and oxygen content in the air is at the highest. If this time is unsuitable, then do so at any time, but only ensure that the stomach is completely empty.

TECHNIQUE

Bhastrika Pranayama

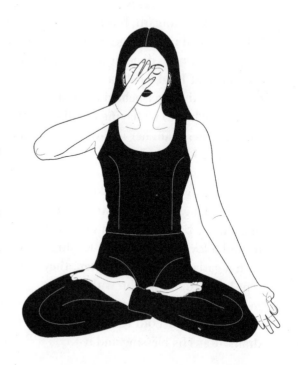

- Sit in *Sukhasana* (The cross legged posture).
- Straighten your back.
- Keep the left hand on left knee in *chin mudra*.
- Place the index and middle finger of the right hand, on the forehead, between the eyebrows.
- Close the right nostril with your thumb.
- Breathe rapidly 20 times through the left nostril with

force, resembling the movement of a bellow.

- Open the right nostril and close the left one with the ring finger.
- Breathe 20 times from this nostril in the same manner.
- Open both the nostrils and breathe from them simultaneously 20 times.
- Inhalation and exhalation should be equal.

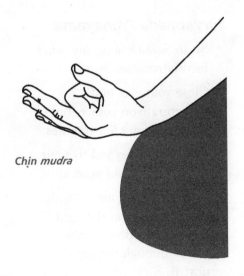

Chin mudra

This is 1 round. Practice 5 rounds in winters and 3 in summer.

Bhastrika is a heating *pranayama* that burns waste and toxins in the body. It strengthens the nervous system and balances the humors (*Kapha* – mucous, *Pitta* – bile, *Vaayu* – gas).

In *Chin mudra*, fingers point up and in *Gyan mudra*, fingers point down.

> NOTE: People with heart ailments, hernia, gastric ulcers, stroke and epilepsy should not do this *pranayama*. Hypertensive people can practice it only after rectifying their condition. (This can be done in seven days with appropriate yogic routine. Please see *Yoga for a Healthy Heart*).

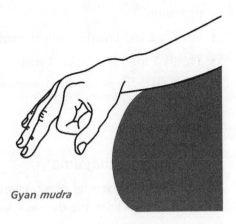

Gyan mudra

Suryabheda Pranayama

- Sit in *Sukhasana* or any other meditative *asana*.

- Close your eyes and concentrate on your natural breathing for a few minutes.

- Open your eyes and fix your gaze on the tip of your nose.

- Closing the left nostril with the ring finger of the right hand, take a deep breath slowly through the right nostril.

- Close both nostrils.

- Bend head to the chest and contract the perineum.

- After a few seconds, relax the perineum.

- Lift head and breathe from the right nostril.

- This is 1 round, practice 3 such rounds.

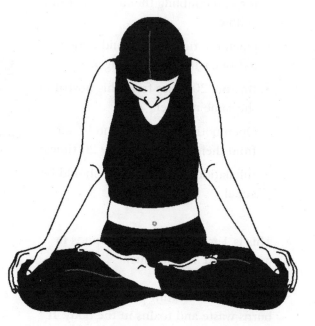

> NOTE: This *pranayama* too generates heat. It should not be done by heart patients, epileptics and people with gastric ulcers.

Nadisodana Pranayama

This is the most essential *pranayama* that is common to all. It purifies the energy pathways ensuring the smooth flow of *prana*.

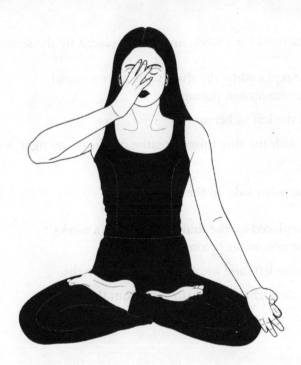

First Stage

- Sit in *Sukhasana* or any other meditative *asana*.

- Straighten your back.

- Keep the left hand on the left knee in *chin mudra*.

- Place the index and middle finger of the right hand on the forehead between the eyebrows.

- Close the right nostril with your thumb.

- Breathe naturally from the left.

- Then closing the left nostril with the ring finger, breathe out from the right.

- Repeat 10 times.

First stage to be practiced for a week, and then replaced by the second stage.

Second stage (to be replaced by the third stage after a week)
- Assume the same *pranayama* posture.
- Breathe in from the left as before.
- Closing the left with the ring finger, breathe out from the right nostril.
- Repeat 10 times.
- Practice from the other side, in the same way.

Third stage (to be replaced by the fourth stage after a week)
- Assume the same posture as before.
- Breathe in from the left, and breathe out from the right.
- Breathe in from the right, and breathe out from the left.
- Repeat 10 times.

> NOTE: This stage and onwards is not meant for heart patients and those with high blood pressure problems.

Fourth and final stage
(Though there are many more advanced stages, this stage will suffice our purpose.)

Assume the same posture and breathe like you have been doing in the third stage, but after inhalation, close both nostrils and retain the breath inside, maintaining the ratio of 1:1:1, meaning the duration of inhalation, retention and exhalation should be the same.

To count both the ratios and the number of rounds, it is convenient to do it in the following manner.

Repeat the number of the round, the desired number of times. Meaning, in the first round, repeat 'one' 5 times or whatever number you are capable of during inhalation. In the same manner, repeat 'one' 5 times during retention and also during exhalation. In the second round, count 'two' 5 times as before.

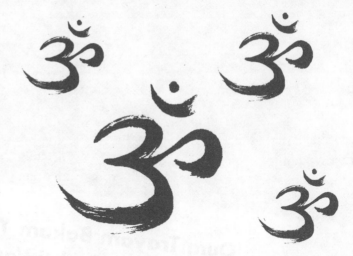

Mantras can also be used for counting instead of the word 'one'. If it is a long *mantra*, repeat once with inhalation, once with retention and once with exhalation. If it is a short one such as *'Oum'*, then it can be added before the number.

For instance,
Oum Oum Oum Oum one,
Oum Oum Oum Oum two.

Gradually increase the number of rounds from 10 to 20 or 25. The duration of inhalation, retention and exhalation also has to be increased gradually by increasing the number of counts from 5 or 7 or to whatever you are comfortable with.

It is said that the *Gayatri Mantra* should be made the unit for counting. This *mantra* is regarded as the source of the *pranic* force and therefore, added to *pranayama*, it can enhance the effect manifold.

Oum Trayam Bakam Yaja Mahe,
Sugandhim Pushti Vardhanam,
Urvaa Rukamiva Bandhanat,
Mrityur Mokshiya Mamvritat

CHAPTER II

MANTRA MAGIC

Mantra Magic

The day Edith Feister was diagnosed with cancer, she met me. Though she was trying to put up a brave front, I could sense her inner turmoil – her voice was shaking, her eyes were dull, and her face was ashen. She was scheduled to fly back to her country, Switzerland, the very next day to undergo the conventional treatment and asked if I could treat her ailment with yoga so that she could avoid the unpleasant medication. I advised her to go ahead and finish the surgery and chemotherapy or else she might have doubts later, but not to take the maintenance dose and instead practice what I was going to teach her. Along with the relevant yogic practices, I taught her a *mantra* and asked her to repeat it mentally whenever possible. In Switzerland, Edith saw the oncologist who explained to her the dreary prognosis of cancer, which according to her would make anybody want to 'jump out of the window and kill oneself'. This depressing meeting was followed by equally depressing tests, which meant hours of confinement and inconvenience. When it was all over, the doctor was amazed to see Edith with no physical signs of stress, which according to him, was most unusual. Edith was repeating the *mantra* throughout.

Mantra is a sound, possessing mystical power. It is said that, with the right *mantra*, even mountains can be moved. The chanting of *mantras* is highly prevalent in India where people use it routinely for various minor and major gains. There are *mantras* for almost everything – money, fame, power, position, spouse, progeny, health, victory in court cases, subjugation of man and animals, and defeating one's enemy – the list is endless.

According to Indian scriptures, *mantra* precedes the Universe. They say that before creation, there was nothing – no form, nor light nor sound – only the Supreme existed in His pure self. In that nothingness, an idea arose in the mind of the Divine to start creation. That single thought caused a vibration, which released a great energy producing the sound of *Oum* – the first *mantra*.

Soon after, *Oum* split into two, then again into fifty different sounds, the permutation and combination of which created this vast universe. The fifty letters of Sanskrit syllables are said to be directly derived from those fifty sounds. Hence, each of its letters is a potential creator, a *mantra*. The combination of specific letters creates a specific *mantra*. It is said that *mantras* were not devised by anybody, but were revealed to the ancient seers during deep meditation when their mind was tuned to the cosmic, absorbing the knowledge therein. The seers kept the knowledge to themselves and passed it on to only a few deserving disciples. Perhaps because incorrectly done or in the wrong hands, such a great power can do more harm then good.

The power of sound, both positive and negative, is not an unknown phenomenon. Soldiers are told to break steps on a bridge, lest the rhythmic sound of their march leads to its collapse. Tibetan lamas are known to gather and disperse clouds by blowing trumpets and beating drums. Nowadays ultrasound is being used to capture the picture of our inner body in great detail. The theory that in the making of Egyptian pyramids, sound manipulation was used to sculpt and lift huge stones may not be so far fetched.

The creative power of sound was demonstrated by Mrs Watta Hughes, a French lady, with an idiophone. This instrument consisted of a hollow tube, a receiver and a flexible membrane on which sand particles were placed. When she sang into the tube, figures such as snakes, stars, flowers and even Virgin Mary with baby Christ in her arms, appeared on the sand. According to the great Guru Swami Satyananda Saraswati, sound can even alter the genetic pattern.

Mantras are seen to affect the human body. American scientists have observed that *mantras* improve cardio vascular, respiratory and endocrinal functions, eliminate stress hormones such as lactate, cortisone and adrenalin from the body and lower serum cholesterol as well as blood pressure. Psychologists, too, have noticed improved scores in emotional stability and neurosis. Research on the *mantra Oum* showed that when 'O' was pronounced, the brain produced alpha waves immediately, and during 'M', the waves changed to theta.

The instantaneous effect of *mantras* can baffle even a non-believer, as I was in my younger days, when an amazing incident took place in our house. A domestic help tripped over a sickle and cut his foot very badly. The gash was big and blood was gushing out. His efforts to stop the bleeding

with a bandage were of no use – the cloth would soak in no time at all. At that moment, my grandmother walked in. She took one look at the man, closed her eyes, muttered something and blew out into the cut. The bleeding stopped in barely five seconds. She does not reveal her *mantra* to anybody and uses it only in dire needs. In India, utmost secrecy is maintained regarding *mantras*. People believe that the gains will be lost if they speak about them.

As *mantras* work on the subtle level, they can affect even from a distance. There was a police officer named Lakshman Mishra in Orissa, an eastern state of India. He was greatly interested in alternative healings. His work took him to the interiors of the province where he came in contact with tribes with extensive knowledge of herbs and *mantras*. He learnt it all from them and has written some wonderful books. He was famous for the *mantra* on snakebites, so much so that whenever a person was bitten by a snake, the relatives would call Mr Mishra who would use his technique to cure the victim.

There are basically two types of *mantras* – *Tantric* and *Vedic*. The *Tantric mantra*, that includes *bija* (seed) works the fastest and the best. But the rituals associated with them are extremely demanding, wherein each step has to be followed with strict precision. If a *mantra* requires one to wear yellow clothes, adorn the idol with yellow sari, offer her yellow flowers and rice, sit on a yellow carpet or a yellow skin, then even the colour orange will not do. Disregarding a rule may even be harmful. Perhaps, because a ritual is meant to tap a specific power centre with its typical colour, sound vibration and other features and any deviation can attract a wrong centre. Therefore, *tantric mantras* should be learnt from a competent Guru directly and practiced under his supervision.

Vedic mantras are benign by nature. They may need some rituals, but are simple and harmless. Some universal *mantras* like *Oum* and *Soham* do not even need that. The best part of these type of *mantras* is that even when mispronounced, they do not harm. There is a very interesting myth about this. In a jungle lived a fearsome dacoit named Ratnakar who killed and robbed travellers for a living. Once Narada, the famed celestial sage, appeared before him and Ratanakar raised his sword to strike. The sage stopped and asked Ratnakar if the latter's family members were willing to share his sin. When Ratnakar replied in the affirmative, Narada suggested the dacoit ascertain it before killing him and Ratnakar agreed to do that. He tied the sage to a tree and went home to put the question before his family. But they refused to comply saying that as a husband and father, it was his duty to provide for his family and how he did that was completely his concern. A distraught Ratnakara returned to the jungle, fell at Narada's feet and begged the sage to save him. Narada taught him the *mantra 'Rama'* and asked him to repeat it whenever possible. Ratnakar sat there and started enchanting the *mantra* and never stopped repeating it. Anthills formed around him but he went on saying *'Rama Rama'* till enlightenment dawned on him. He became a great sage and came to be known as Rishi Valmiki, who is said to have written the great Indian epic, *Ramayana*. The interesting part of this story is that Ratnakara could not say *'Rama Rama'* in the beginning, but *'Mara Mara'* which means 'died, died'.

Rama is a simple universal *mantra* used for divine protection against all calamities. Though it is the name of an Indian god, the *mantra 'Rama'* has nothing to do with the Hindu religion. *Mantras* were based on appropriate sound vibrations with specific forms. Rather, the names and forms of deities are said to have evolved on the basis of these *mantras*.

The *mantra 'Rama'* can either be spoken or written down. The latter is supposed to be more effective than the former one. Traditionally, on certain auspicious days, *'Rama'* is written with vermilion on the leaves of a particular tree called *bel*, which are then offered to lord Shiva. (*Bel* leaves have therapeutic value and have a positive toning effect on the liver.) People who cannot practice the other *mantras* for some reason can benefit greatly from this simple one.

A *mantra* which is specifically used by many to cure all ailments including cancer is the *Dhanwantari Mantra*. It should be repeated as instructed till the disease is cured, but not less than six months. In addition, all cancer patients should recite *Mahamritunjaya Mantra* – literally meaning 'the death defying *mantra*' and this was the one I had taught Edith. *Mahamritunjaya Mantra* is supposed to bestow longevity to its practitioner. In India, people often turn to this *mantra* when their life is in danger. Usually priests conduct the chanting for the affected person, of course, for a price. Depending on the individual's financial capacity, the number of *mantras* to be chanted and that of priests are fixed beforehand. If the person wants one lakh *mantra* repetition in a hundred days, everyday it has to be chanted one thousand times, which can be accomplished by ten priests in less than an hour – each reciting the minimum required number of a hundred and eight times – or by one priest in six to seven hours. At my Guruji's ashram in Munger, Bihar, often disciples from all over the world send requests for *Mahamritunjaya Mantra* to be repeated for a particular person and on Saturdays, it is conducted free of cost by the yogis and inmates with wonderful results. But it is not mandatory to get it done by others – the sufferer can do it her/himself. Friends and family members may join if they so wish.

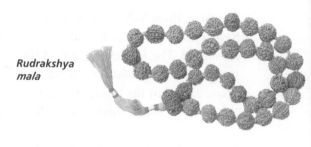

Rudrakshya mala

A *mantra* can be repeated mentally, loudly or even whispered or one can also combine all the methods. It should be repeated one hundred and eight times at one go, though people do benefit by repeating it fifty-four times or even twenty-seven times in three to four sessions everyday. Use a *mala* or rosary beads to count the number. The material used for making the beads or rosary also generate energy and hence, the *mala* is chosen according to the *mantra*.

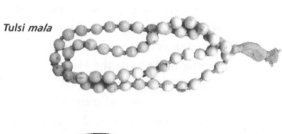

Tulsi mala

Rudrakshya is used for *Mahamrutunjaya Mantra* while *tulsi* (basil) can be used for *Dhanwantari*. There is a particular way to use the *mala* – the thumb and the ring finger of the right hand should be used to hold it, while the middle finger

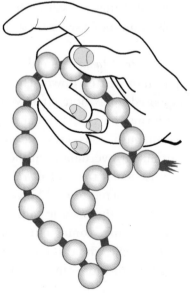

should rotate the beads. It can also be hung from the last three fingers joined together. Ideally, the hand is kept in front of the heart with the arms raised to free the armpit. This position can get quite uncomfortable. To get relief many use a wooden support for the arm.

A *mantra* should be practiced in an allotted room or a corner, which is airy and quiet. Once chosen, the place should not be changed, as it retains the vibration of the *mantra* and helps calm the practitioner, the moment she/he sits down. There should not be any pictures of unhappiness, turbulence or violence on the walls. If possible hang a few pictures of gods and saints.

TECHNIQUE

- After bathing, spread a small rug.
- Light a lamp or *diya* and burn incense.
- Place a **Mahamritunjaya Yantra** in front – a *yantra* is a pictorial form of a *mantra*.
- Calm your mind, close your eyes and steady the body.
- Practice deep breathing for a few minutes.

Mahamrityunjaya Yantra

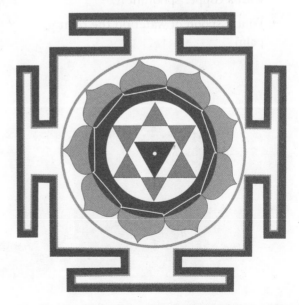

- Say the purpose of the repetition and number of the *mantra* in your mind.

Hold the rosary.

Start the *mantra*.

Mahmrityunjaya Mantra

Oum Trayam Bakam Yaja Mahe,
Sugandhim Pushti Vardhanam,
Urvaa Rukamiva Bandhanat,
Mrityur Mokshiya Mamvritat.

The following ritual should precede **Dhanwantri Mantra**:

- Take a little water in a copper glass with a copper spoon in it.
- Pour 1 spoon of water on the right palm.

- Say **Oum Achyta Namah** and put the water in your mouth without your hand touching your lips.
- Pour another spoon of water and say **Oum Anantaya Namah** and drink the water.
- The third time, say, **Oum Govindaya Namah.**

Dhanwantari Mantra

Oum Namah Bhagavate,
Dhanwantaraye, amrita kalasha hastaya,
Sarvaamaya Vinashaaya,
Trailokyanathaaya
Shri Maha Vishnave swaha.

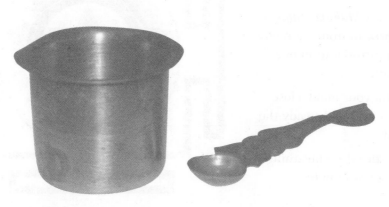

Some *mantras*:

Oum Namah Shivaya
Hari Oum
Amen
Amin
Arhint
Vahe Guru
Asham Vohu
Oum Mani Padme Hum

Universal *mantras*
Oum
Soham (I am that)
Aham Brahmasmi (I am consciousness)
Tat Twan Asi (You are that)

CHAPTER III

YAGNYA OR THE SACRIFICIAL FIRE

Yagnya or the Sacrificial Fire

Though yoga has nothing to do with *yagnya*, many say that a *mantra's* efficacy is enhanced when *yagnya* or sacrificial fire, is performed. It is said that a *mantra* for health eliminates toxic negative energy from the body, which is consumed and destroyed for good by the fire in front.

Yagnya occupied the most important position in the Vedic life. The Vedas are the ancient scriptures of India, which take their name from *vidya,* meaning knowledge. True to their meaning, these scriptures contain truth regarding all aspects of the universe – its origin, nature, content, science, alchemy, topography as well as its animate and inanimate objects. It is said that, all that has already been known and all that which will ever be known are contained in the Vedas. The profoundness of Vedic knowledge has baffled all and sundry. For instance, thousands of years before science discovered the earth to be round and that it goes around the sun, Vedas had proclaimed it.

In India, the Vedic words are considered the ultimate and in the past, its recommendations were never discarded. People followed them unquestioningly. They led their lives in accordance with the Vedas, which were supposed to fulfill all their desires – material as well as spiritual, and in the end leave the world with contentment. The Vedas had classified human desires into four:

1. *Artha* or wealth
2. *Dharma* or proficiency in one's chosen line of work
3. *Kama* or passion
4. *Mokshya* or liberation

In order to achieve these systematically, the Vedas had divided the lifespan of an individual – which was supposed to be a hundred years according to these scriptures – into four phases, and a specific lifestyle was recommended for each phase.

The first quarter was to be spent in the Guru's abode and acquire professional skills as well as spiritual knowledge. The second phase, which began at the age of twenty-five years, was meant to fulfill all the material desires without neglecting the worldly duties. In the third quarter, people were expected to withdraw from active life and retire to the jungle to pursue spiritual goals. They were supposed to lead a simple life and look after their own needs. During this phase, people did not cut off their social ties and returned to their families intermittently. But in the last twenty-five years or till their death, they were required to renounce the world completely and live alone in a hut. This speaks volumes of their physical and mental superiority. To live away from home, hospital, doctors and an attendant at that age is unthinkable for people of today. The Vedic routine followed by people in ancient times must be greatly responsible for their extraordinary strength, endurance and courage.

Yagnya was the central practice of the Vedic routine. The main features of a *yagnya* are *mantras*, the fire and the oblations or offerings that go into it. The beneficial effects of a *yagnya* have now been scientifically established. For instance, the vapour produced by burning various materials, has medicinal properties that cure many ailments of the performer and the onlooker. One of the common *yagnya*, which everybody is recommended to perform twice a day is the *Gayatri*. It is believed that, apart from bestowing the right knowledge, it energises the body and eliminates all diseases. The *mantra* is also said to negate the ill effects of disharmonious and destructive sounds that attack an individual from various sources. Cancer patients can benefit greatly by performing this *yagnya*. This should be performed in the morning and *Mahamritunjaya Yagnya* in the evening.

The procedure for *yagnya* is rather elaborate but nowadays learned priests have shortened the *Gayatri Yagnya* for the benefit of ordinary people. It is argued that, this *mantras* is so powerful that by simply reciting it, one can attain the desired objectives. With the fire in front, it can be infallible and the other paraphernalia can be dispensed with.

Gayatri Yagnya: the necessary steps

- After taking a bath in the morning, ideally at sunrise, spread a small rug on the floor with the sealed edges towards the north and the south.
- Sit facing the north.
- Place the *yagnya* pot in front with a few pieces of firewood in it.
- Keep some *ghee* (clarified butter) and a long spoon in a vessel.
- To count the number of *mantras*, keep 108 beads in a cup and a plate to hold the counted ones.
- Keep some water in a copper glass with a copper spoon in it.
- Take a spoonful of water in your right hand and cover it with your left hand.
- Repeat the *Gayatri Mantra* 3 times mentally and state the purpose of doing the *yagnya* and sprinkle the water around you.

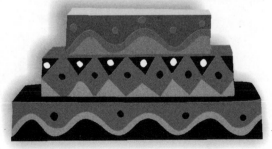

A traditional *havan kund* is made of earthen bricks and is decorated with *alpana*.

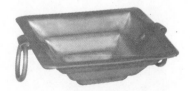

A smaller *havan kund* made of copper for home worship.

Om Bhurbhuvah Swaha
Tatsavitur varenyam
Bhargo devasya dhee mahidhiyo
Yonah prachodayat.

- Practice the second stage of *Nadisodana Pranayama* 8 times, but only in 1 direction, that is, inhale from the left and exhale from the right.

- Concentrate on the naval centre during inhalation, on the heart centre during retention and on the eyebrow centre during exhalation.

- Practice the following *mudras* and gestures as shown in the pictures one after the other.

- These *mudras* connect the *prana* of the body with the cosmic one and ensure its smooth flow in the physical plane.

Gayatri Yantra

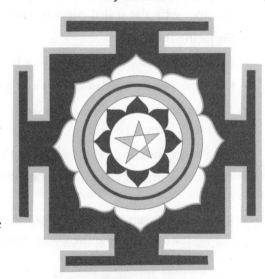

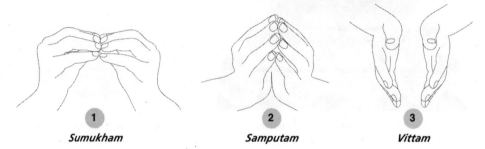

1	2	3
Sumukham	**Samputam**	**Vittam**

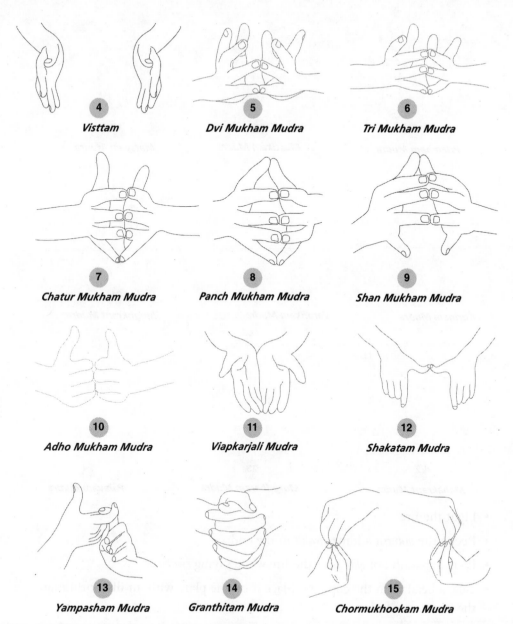

4
Visttam

5
Dvi Mukham Mudra

6
Tri Mukham Mudra

7
Chatur Mukham Mudra

8
Panch Mukham Mudra

9
Shan Mukham Mudra

10
Adho Mukham Mudra

11
Viapkarjali Mudra

12
Shakatam Mudra

13
Yampasham Mudra

14
Granthitam Mudra

15
Chormukhookam Mudra

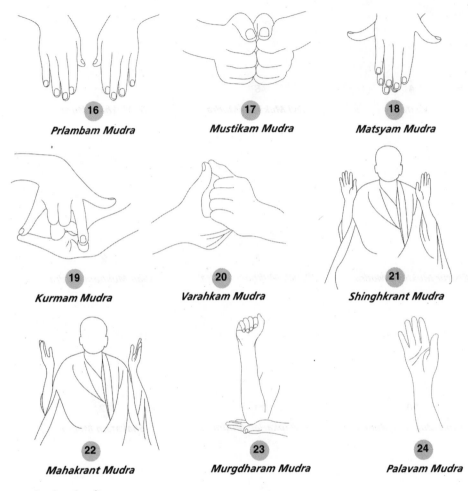

16 Prlambam Mudra

17 Mustikam Mudra

18 Matsyam Mudra

19 Kurmam Mudra

20 Varahkam Mudra

21 Shinghkrant Mudra

22 Mahakrant Mudra

23 Murgdharam Mudra

24 Palavam Mudra

- Light the fire.
- Recite the *mantra* adding *swaha* in the end.
- Pour a spoonful of *ghee* into the fire while saying *swaha*.
- Take a bead from the cup, and place it on the plate without discontinuing the *mantra* recitation.

- Continue the process till the cup of beads is empty.
- Practice the following *mudras*.

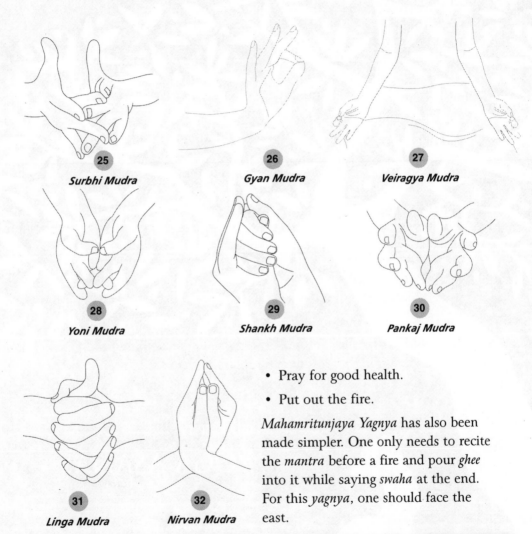

25 Surbhi Mudra

26 Gyan Mudra

27 Veiragya Mudra

28 Yoni Mudra

29 Shankh Mudra

30 Pankaj Mudra

31 Linga Mudra

32 Nirvan Mudra

- Pray for good health.
- Put out the fire.

Mahamritunjaya Yagnya has also been made simpler. One only needs to recite the *mantra* before a fire and pour *ghee* into it while saying *swaha* at the end. For this *yagnya*, one should face the east.

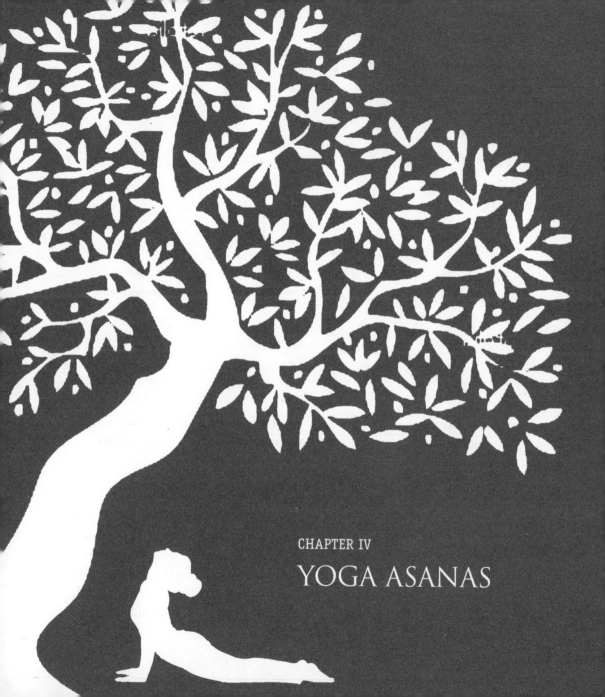

CHAPTER IV

YOGA ASANAS

Yoga Asanas

According to yoga every cell in the body needs *prana* to live and function. There are seventy-two thousand energy channels called *nadis* that carry *prana* to reach each cell. These *nadis* are of two types – *ida* and *pingala*. Though the same energy flows in both the *nadis*, the characteristics in each are different from the other.

The *ida* current is described as blue, feminine, cool and passive, while *pingala* current is red, hot, masculine and dynamic. *Ida* is connected with the right hemisphere of the brain and energises the mental activities, while *pingala* is connected with the left hemisphere and energises physical activities. Generally, only one *nadi* is active at any given time. To determine which *nadi* is active, one needs to check the flow of breath. If it is through the left nostril, *ida* is

active; and if the right is flowing, *pingala* is functioning. The *nadis* work alternately for forty-five minutes to one hour in good health and maintain balance in the functioning of all the physical and mental faculties. When one *nadi* is active much in excess than the other one, it indicates ill health and is actually the outcome of a faulty lifestyle. Incorrect food, excessive excitement, stress, lack of rest, and inadequate physical activities can create blockages in the energy pathways, disrupting the *pranic* flow. This leads to unequal distribution of *prana* to the body tissues, leading to collection of *prana* at certain places, while other parts have less of it. The deprived cells are bound to become weak and diseased.

That one nostril breathing leads to ailments was observed by Dr Riga, an

ENT specialist. Many of his patients who breathed mostly through the left nostril due to some structural obstruction in the nose had respiratory ailments such as sinusitis, pharyngitis, laryngitis, bronchitis and tonsillitis. The other diseases these people suffered from were headache, hyper thyroidism, heart problems, malfunctioning liver, gastritis, colitis, ulcers, constipation and reproductive system ailments. Those who breathe mostly through the right nostril, generally, suffered from high blood pressure. Most interestingly, he found that when the patient's nasal problems were rectified, the other diseases also disappeared.

To remove *pranic* blockages, the main reason for single nostril breathing, *yoga asana* or yogic postures are the most effective way. *Asanas* affect the body very deeply and should not be regarded as physical exercises. In appearance, both forms may be similar, but in effect, they are much different. The most glaring example in ordinary physical exercises is that, the body's oxygen consumption becomes very high, while during *yoga asnas*, it

decreases greatly. This indicates that, even though the body is actively working during yoga, it is relaxed.

Asanas are even more relaxing than normal rest. Tests have shown that while a man was lying on the bed, his body still retained twenty units of tension. But when he practiced *yoga asana*, the tension level dropped dramatically. It might seem unbelievable, but in *Bhujangasana*, the tension at the lower back measured zero.

Secondly, while exercises mainly affect the muscles and bones, yoga has been found to affect the finer functioning of the nervous system and the glandular system. The added advantage of the dynamic *asanas* is that they fulfill the needs of normal aerobic exercises.

Any form of physical exercise is essential for good health, not only because they tone up the muscles and improve blood circulation, but also because they raise the level of serotonin in the brain. This chemical is a neuro-transmitter, which stimulates the production of Endomorphine. But only the right amount of exercise is beneficial. Over exercising taxes the heart and weakens immunity and too little of it has no value. In yoga, one cannot go wrong as the all-knowing ancient *yogis* have specified the number of each practice.

Yoga asanas are so powerful that their effect is felt almost immedietely. I remember this gentleman, a Swedish diplomat who used to attend my class in the evening. He would come in quite tired, flop on the yoga mat and not even stir for some time; then, would pull himself up and start practicing the *asanas*. Initially, his movements would be absolutely lifeless, but by the end of the session, he would be smiling and joking. He would feel so energetic that he preferred to walk back to his house, which was at least five kilometres away.

The *asanas* must be chosen correctly to cure an ailment as it is obvious that, an *asana* for the back cannot cure migraine. Many continue to suffer from diseases inspite of practicing yoga for years. Maybe, it is because they choose the wrong ones or practice them incorrectly.

Cancer is considered an outcome of a weak eliminative system and therefore *asanas* that strengthen the liver, intestine and skin, should become the focus, but the ones that remove the *pranic* blockages should also be included. The following are the *asanas* to do just that.

Leg Rotation (Single)

- Lie down on your back.
- Lift the right leg 6 inches above the ground.
- Rotate the leg 5 times clockwise and 5 times anti-clockwise.

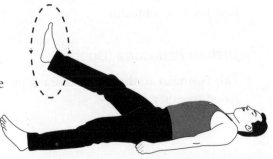

- Bring the leg down to the ground.
- Repeat with the left leg.

Rest in *Shavasana* for 4 or 5 breaths.

Leg Rotation (Double)

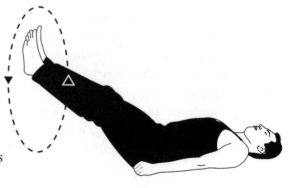

- Lift both legs together and rotate them 5 times clockwise and 5 times anti-clockwise.

Rest for 4 or 5 breaths.

Utthan Padasana (Single)

- Lift the right leg without bending the knee to a vertical position.
- Hold for a few seconds.
- Slowly bring the leg down to the ground.
- Repeat 5 times.
- Repeat with the left leg.

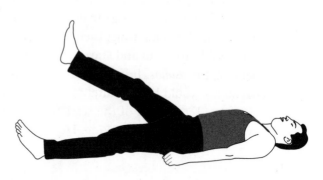

Rest for 4 or 5 breaths.

Utthan Padasana (Double)

This is similar to the previous *asana* but in this *asana* both the legs have to be raised together.

Naukasana

- Lie down on your back.
- Take a deep breath.
- Lift up your trunk, legs and arms simultaneously, 10-12 inches above the ground. The head, hands and feet should be at the same level.
- Hold the posture for as long as you can hold your breath.
- Exhaling, come down.

After 2-3 breaths, practice again. Repeat 5 times.

Surya Namaskar

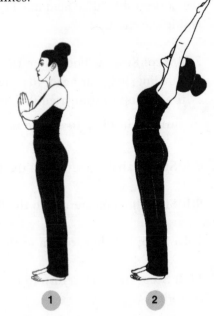

1st Step: Stand straight with feet together and hands folded to a *'namaskar'* (greeting gesture) and hold in front of the chest.

2nd Step: Inhaling, lift arms above you. Turn face upward to stretch the neck, and bend a little backward.

3rd Step: Exhaling, bend forward.
- Place the hands on the floor a little in front and outside the feet.

- You may bend the knees initially if necessary.

4th Step: Inhaling, extend the left leg all the way back.
- Bring the hips down.
- The right knee should be pointing forward.
- Turn the face up.

5th Step: Exhaling, lift the bottom up.
- Take the right foot back to join the left one.
- Put the head in between the arms (do not disturb the position of the hands).

6th Step: Holding the breath out, lower your body to rest on the ground but the bottom should be held up. The hands should remain beside the chest.

7th Step: Rest the bottom on the floor.
- Inhaling, lift your head, the chest and the stomach all the way up to straighten the arms.
- Turn the head up to stretch the neck well.

8th Step: Exhaling, return to the fifth position.

9th Step: Inhaling, return to the fouth position.

10th Step: Exhaling, return to the third position.

11th Step: Inhaling, return to the second position.

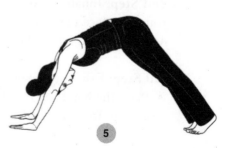

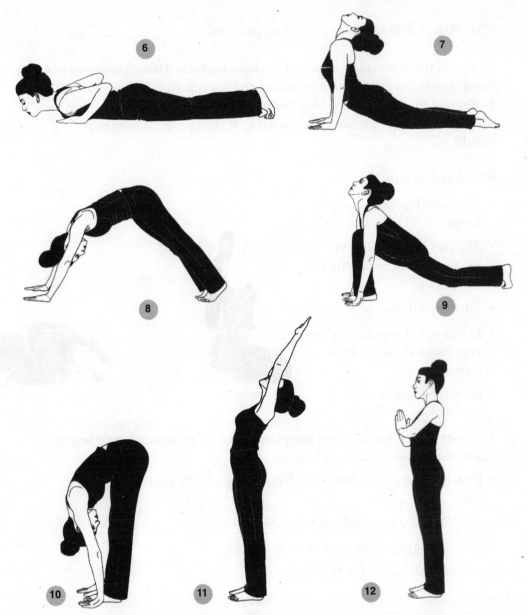

12th Step: Exhaling, return to the first position.

Repeat on the other side, i.e. extend the right leg back. These 2 cycles form 1 round. Practice 6 to 12 rounds according to your capacity. You can start with 3 or even 1 round. After finishing the desired number of rounds, lie down in *Shavasana* till your breathing is normal (i.e. at the rate of 10 breaths per round.)

Shashankasana

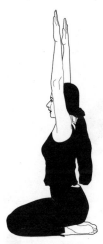
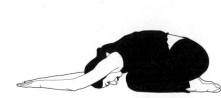

- Fold your legs and sit on the heels.

- The toes should touch but the feet should not overlap each other.

- Inhaling, lift your arms up.

- Exhaling and maintaining the position of the arms, bend forward.

- Keep the forearms and forehead on the ground.

- If your body is too stiff, you can place a cushion underneath your bottom and also separate the knees initially.

- Breathe normally. Starting with 5 breaths, gradually increase them to a 100.

- Inhaling, raise your body and the arms.

- Exhaling, bring the arms down to the thighs.

Lie down in *Shavasana* for 10 breaths.

Shavasana

- Lie down on your back in a straight line with the legs around 18 inches apart.

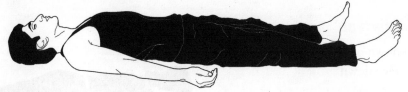

- Move hands a little away from the body with the palms facing up.
- Close your eyes.
- Breathe naturally.
- Count breaths backward.
- 10 breaths.

Bhujangasana

- Lie down on your stomach.
- Keep hands flat on the ground and away from the chest.
- Inhaling, turn the face up and rise to straighten the arms.
- Bend head backward to stretch the neck.
- The back should be well-arched with the lower abdomen on the ground.
- Hold the posture for as long as you are comfortable.

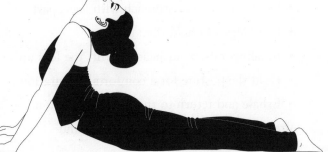

- Exhaling, return to the starting position.

Repeat this process by starting with 1 round and then gradually increase it to 5 rounds.

Shalabhasana

- Lie down on your stomach with the face down.
- Place hands under the thighs with palms facing down.
- Inhale.
- Holding the breath in, lift legs together without bending the knees.
- Hold the posture for as long as comfortable.
- Exhaling, bring the legs down.

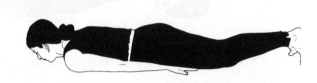

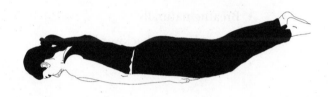

After a short rest of 2-3 breaths, repeat by starting with 1 round and then increase it to 5 rounds.

Dhanurasana

- Lie down on your stomach with legs apart.
- Bend legs and hold the ankles.
- Inhaling, raise your head and lift the legs up.
- Hold the posture for a comfortable duration.
- Exhale and return to the starting position.

After 2-3 breaths, repeat the process and practice 3 rounds.

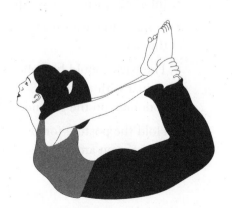

Paschimottanasana

- Sit down with legs extended in front.
- Raise your arms straight up.
- Inhale.
- Exhaling, bend forward and hold your toes.
- If that is not possible, hold your ankles or even your calves.
- Breathe naturally.

Starting with 5 breaths gradually increase it to 20.

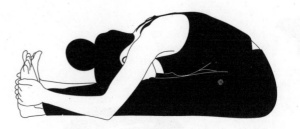

Kandhrasana

- Lie down on your back.
- Bend legs and place the feet outside the hips.
- Hold your ankles.
- Inhaling, lift your pelvis.
- Hold the posture for a comfortable duration.
- Exhaling, come down.
- Repeat 3 times.

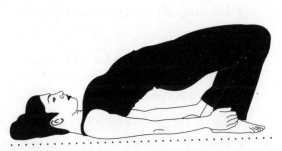

Pranamasana

- Fold your legs underneath and sit on your heels.
- Grasp your calves.
- Exhaling, bend forward and keep your forehead on the ground.

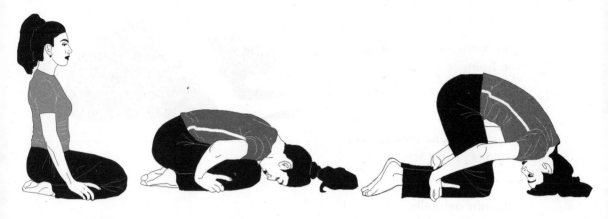

- Lift your hips up while rolling the head so that when you are fully raised, the weight of the body falls on the corner of the head and not on the top.

- Hold the posture for as long as comfortable.

- Roll back the head while lowering your body to the heels.

- Inhaling, lift your head and sit up.

- Exhale.

Lie down in *Shavasana* for 10 breaths.

Ardhamatsyendrasana

- Sit on the ground with legs stretched in front.

- Bend the right leg and keep the right heel beside the left hip.

- The knee should be pointing straight ahead.

- Bend the left leg and place the left foot flat on the ground in front of the right knee.

- Take the right arm to the left.

- Hitching the right arm with the left knee, hold the left ankle with the right hand.
- Straighten your body and take a breath.
- Exhaling, turn to your left, twisting the body and the head as far as possible without putting any undue strain.
- Breathe naturally 20 times.
- Inhaling, twist back to the former position
- Change legs and practice on the right side

Lie down in *Shavasana* for 10 breaths.

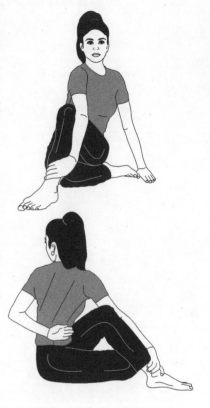

People with heart ailments including high blood-pressure should not practice any of these *asanas* except *Shashankasana* and *Shavasana*. They should first normalise their blood-pressure, which can be done easily in a week with the right yoga. Backache sufferers can practice *Shashankasana, Bhujangasana, Shalabhasana, Dhanurasana, Kandhrasana* and *Ardhamatsyendrasana*.

They should follow the routine contained in the book. However, it is advisable to learn directly from a yoga expert.

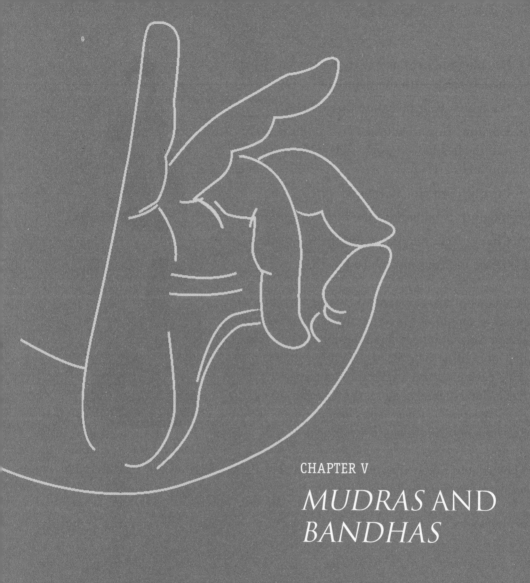

CHAPTER V

MUDRAS AND *BANDHAS*

Mudras and *Bandhas*

In a world where everything is in state of flux, so is *prana*. It enters the body, flows in to nourish the cells and leaves. Often, during illnesses, the outflow can be more than the inflow, which can hinder cure and for optimal use, its escape needs to be prevented. Yoga has four postures called *bandhas* to do just that. The literal meaning of *bandha* is lock as well as dam. It is not enough to lock the *prana* in, but it should be locked in the right places. Each *bandha* is entrusted to hold the *prana* in a specific area.

According to the functions, the *pranic* body is divided into five parts and so is the *prana*. Each sub *prana* occupies a specific part and carries out specific functions. When these functions are disturbed, it indicates depletion of *prana* in that area.

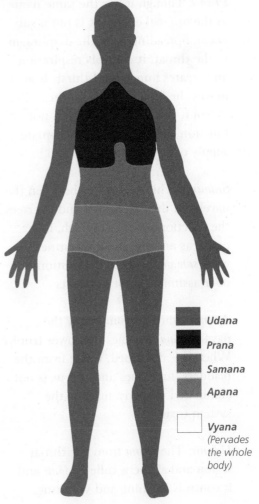

Udana

Prana

Samana

Apana

Vyana
(Pervades the whole body)

These five sub-*pranas* are: 1. *Samana*;
2. *Udana*; 3. *Prana*; 4. *Apana;* and
5. *Vyana*

Prana: Though it has the same name as the original energy, it is but a sub *prana*. Spreading from the diaphragm to the throat, it controls respiration and creates hunger and thirst. It also moves the food down from the gullet. When it is weak, the lungs do not function well leading to inadequate supply of oxygen to the system.

Samana: This energy lies between the navel and the diaphragm and oversees the functions of the stomach, liver, pancreas and the small intestines. A weak *samana* leads to indigestion or poor assimilation of nutrients.

Apana: Starting from below the naval, *apana* occupies the lower trunk. When it is disturbed, waste from the bladders, intestines and uterus is not eliminated properly, making the system toxic.

Udana: The *prana* from the throat region and above is called *udana* and it controls belching and vomiting.

When it is weak, gas from the stomach cannot escape through the mouth and gives the feeling of bloating.

Vyana: The rest of the body, mainly the limbs, fall under *vyana*. A weak *vyana* leads to improper circulation of blood and lymph.

Of the three main *bandhas, Jalandhar* is meant for the upper part of the body, *Udiyana* for the mid-trunk and *Moola* for the lower trunk. *Maha Bandha,* which is the combination of all the three *bandhas,* affects the entire body and in a magnified way.

Mudras direct the energy to specific parts of the body. These practices can be postures, hand gestures or a body part position. Of these, *Chin Mudra, Gyan Mudra* and *Vajaroli* are used extensively in yoga. The former two *mudras* re-direct the escaping *prana* inwards, while *Vajaroli* is known to stimulate the *kundalini* – the store house of *prana* in the body. A few sparks from it is said to energise the body as nothing else can.

Jalandhara Bandha

- Sit in *Padmasana* – the lotus pose.
- Keep your hands on the knees.
- Take a deep breath.
- Bend your head till the chin is pressed against the chest (called chin lock).
- By lifting the shoulder, straighten your arms (called shoulder lock).
- Hold the posture till you can retain your breath comfortably.
- Release the shoulder lock by dropping the shoulder; lift your head up.
- Exhale.

Wait till your breathing becomes normal, and then practice again.

Repeat 5 times.

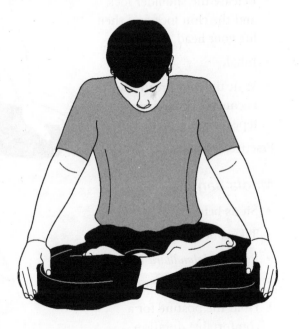

Uddiyana Bandha

- Sit in the lotus pose with hands on the knees.
- Take a deep breath.
- Pucker your lips.
- Exhaling, from the mouth bend your head down to do a chin lock and then a shoulder lock.

- Pull in your stomach as much as possible.
- Hold the posture for a comfortable duration.
- Relax your stomach.
- Release the shoulder lock and the chin lock and then lift your head.
- Inhale.
- Wait till your breathing becomes normal before repeating.

Practice 5 rounds.

Moola Bandha

- Sit as before.
- Take a deep breath.
- Practice *Jalandhara Bandha*.
- Contract your perineum.
- Hold the posture for a comfortable duration.
- Relax the perineum.
- Release the shoulder lock and the chin lock.
- Exhale.

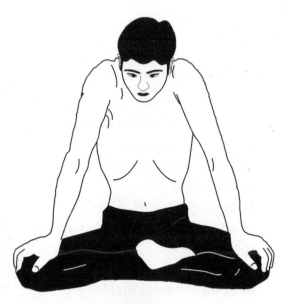

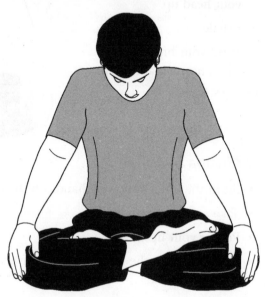

- After your breathing becomes normal, practice again.

Repeat 5 times.

Maha Bandha

Combine 3 *bandhas* i.e. first practice *Uddiyana Bandha*, and then contract the perinium.

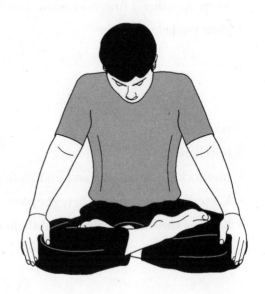

Chin Mudra

- Bend the index finger and touch the base of the thumb lightly.
- Keep the other 3 fingers relaxed and slightly apart from another.
- Turn the palm up.

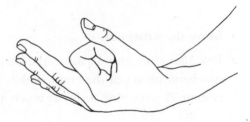

Gyana Mudra

- Touch the tip of the thumb with the index finger.
- Keep the other 3 fingers separate and relaxed.
- Turn the palm down.

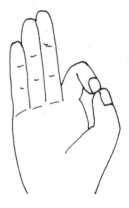

Yoni Mudra

- Join hands.
- Interlock the little, ring and middle fingers.
- Keep the index fingers where they are.
- Keeping the thumbs joined, pull them towards your body to be completely stretched.

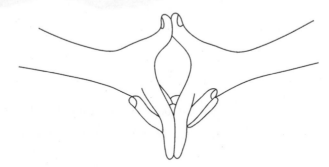

- Move the wrists out.
- *Yoni Mudra* not only balances the energies in the body, it also balances the two hemispheres of the brain, which helps in rectifying the faults of the system. Practice this *mudra* as much as possible.

Vajroli

- Sit in *Vajrasana*.
- Contract the muscles as you do to control urination.
- Hold for 10 counts.
- Release the contraction.
- Repeat 50 times.

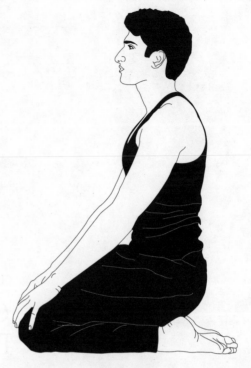

Vajrasana

CHAPTER VI

CHAKRA PURIFICATION

Chakra Purification

The *pranic* body is composed of not only *nadis* and *prana,* but also energy centres called *chakras*. These swirling masses of energy that resemble lotus flowers with the petals representing the outlets of *prana,* vibrate with a specific frequency and produce specific sounds. There are innumerable *chakras* in our body, but the ones located on the spinal column are the vital ones. In yoga, these *chakras* occupy prime positions because of the important functions they perform. They:

a) store *prana*
b) regulate proper distribution of energy
c) provide the connection between *kundalini* and the higher brain centres.

In most people, only one-tenth part of the brain functions and it has not yet been discovered what the other nine-tenth area contains. This non-functioning part is called the 'silent area'.

According to yoga, many unknown higher faculties are present in this area. With evolution, when *kundalini* becomes active naturally, in everybody, all these centres will be automatically operational. Till then they remain dormant But, with yoga, it is possible to activate them even now. The secret lies in the *chakras*

To reach the core of the *chakras* where the switches for the dormant centres lie, the *chakras* needs to be first purified. Often, impurities in the body and mind make a *chakra* sluggish, its frequency and velocity becomes lower, the sound it produces becomes disharmonious and the *pranic* flow around it gets disturbed. This causes malfunction of glands and organs it controls. When the *chakra* is purified, the resultant diseases disappear. No means may cure a disease unless the fault in the *chakra* is corrected. Thus, if not for the higher purposes, *chakras* should be purified to attain perfect health which can be achieved through *mantras,* music, meditation or concentration, on any one of the aspects of the *chakras* such as its form, element, location, deity, sound and colour.

The six major *chakras* are:

Mooladhara Chakra

It is the lowest *chakra*, located near the cocygal plexus, the exact location in the male body is the perineum, while in the female body, it is the cervix. It is a dark red coloured lotus, with four petals. One of the following Sanskrit syllables, *wam, sham, ssham, sam* is written on each petal. In the flower is a yellow square, surrounded by eight golden spears. Inside the square is an elephant with seven trunks. In the centre of the square and above the elephant is an inverted triangle of deep

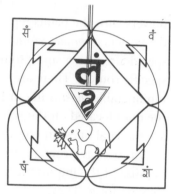

red colour within which is a gray smoky coloured *Shivalingam*, with a snake coiled around it three and a half times. On top of the triangle, is a *bija mantra* (seed) of this *chakra-lam*. The musical note that it responds to is 'Sa' ('Do' in western music). The presiding deities of *Mooladhara* are Lord Ganesh and Goddess Dakini and its element is Earth. *Mooladhara* controls the excretory and reproductive organs, and also the excretion of reproductive hormones in this region. It is also connected with the nose and the sense of smell. People with awakened *Mooladhara* become adept at learning and remain ever cheerful and free from diseases.

Swadhistan Chakra

About one and a half inch above *Mooladhara*, at the base of the spinal column, corresponding to the sacral nerve plexus is *Swadishtan chakra*. This lotus has six orange-red petals, each carrying a letter from – *bam, bham, mam, yam, ram* and *lam*. Inside the flower, is a crescent shape moon formed by two circles. In the moon is a crocodile and on it is the *bija mantra, wam*, in white. The element of *Swadhishtan* is water and responds to the musical note 'Re'. The presiding deities of this *chakra* are Lord Vishnu and Goddess Rakini. *Swadhishtan* controls the reproductive glands and organs and is connected with the sense of taste.

Manipura Chakra

Directly behind the naval, on the spinal column, is *Manipura Chakra*, which corresponds to the solar plexus. The ten petals of this *chakra* are bright yellow, and the letters on the petals are *dum, dhum, num, tam, tham dam, dham, nam, pum, pham* in blue. Inside the lotus is a red inverted triangle and on the lower side of the triangle, is a ram on which appears the *bija mantra* as *ram*. Its element is fire and is connected with the eyes. Its corresponding note is *Ga(mi) Manipura* controls digestion and assimilation.

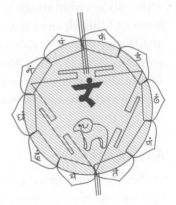

Anahata Chakra

On the spinal column behind the heart, corresponding the cardiac plexus, is the *Anahata chakra*. It has twelve blue petals and the inscribed letters on them are *kam, kham, gam, gham, ang, cam, cham, jam, jham, nyam, tam, tham*. In the middle, there are two interlaced triangles which appear like a hexagon. Inside the hexagon is a black antelope, above which is present the *bija mantra, yam*.

The element of *Anahata* is air and it is associated with the hands and the sense of touch. Heart, lungs and the thymus glands are controlled by this *chakra*.

Visuddhi Chakra

This *chakra* corresponds with the cervical plexus and is located behind the throat. It is a purple coloured lotus with sixteen petals and Sanskrit vowels appear on the petals. Inside the lotus is a white circle within which is a white elephant. The *mantra* of this element is *ham*, its element is ether and the musical note to stimulate it is *'pa'*. The presiding deity is *Sada Shiva* and Goddess *Sakini*. This *chakra* is connected with the ear and sense of hearing and controls the functions of the thyroid and the throat.

Agya Chakra

At the top of the spinal column is *Agya Chakra* with two silvery gray lotus petals, one has the sun, and the other, carries the moon. Inside the lotus is a circle and in it is an inverted triangle. This *chakra's Bija Mantra* is *'Oum'*, which is present inside the triangle. At the bottom of the circle is a black *Shiva Lingam* and its deity is *Param Shaiva*.

Apart from concentrating on the attributes of a *chakra* to stimulate it, *Chakra Shuddhi* meditation

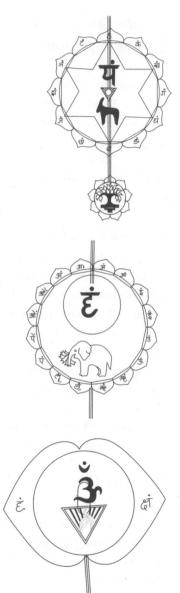

should be done for seven to eight minutes to purify them all. Also, *Trataka* should be done to energise the *Agyan Chakra* as this *chakra* controls all other *chakras*.

TECHNIQUE

Trataka

- Sit in a cross-legged posture, keeping the back straight.
- At an arm's distance, place a lit candle on a stand in front of you. (The flame should be at eye level.)
- Close your eyes and still your body.
- Concentrate on your natural breath for 2-3 minutes.
- Open your eyes and look at the brightest spot in the candle flame.

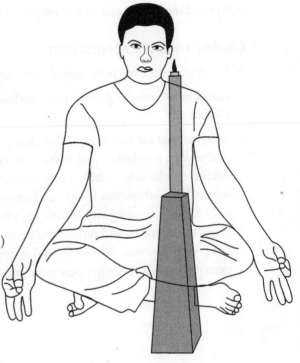

- Without blinking, gaze steadily for half a minute or so (close your eyes before they start to water).
- Close your eyes gently.
- You will see the after image before the closed eyes. Concentrate on that image till it fades.
- Imagine the flame on the same spot in your closed eyes and continue concentrating on it for 7-8 minutes.
- Open your eyes.

Once you become familiar with the technique, keep the symbol of the concerned *chakra* instead of the candle. This is *Trataka*.

Chakra Shuddhi Meditation

- Sit in a meditative pose and close your eyes. Maintain a still posture.

- Concentrate on the point in the abdomen just in front of *Swadhishtan Chakra*.

- Imagine you are breathing from that point. Your breath goes straight to this *chakra* with inhalation and comes out from the abdomen with exhalation. After a few breaths, add it's *bija mantra*, *'vam'* to your breath and mentally repeat *'vam'* when you inhale and again repeat it when you exhale. Practice it 27 times, counting the breath backwards. After you reach one, shift your focus to the naval and repeat the process with *Manipura Chakra*. Do the same with *Anahata, Vishuddhi* and *Agyan*. Take your mind away from external sounds. Slowly open your eyes.

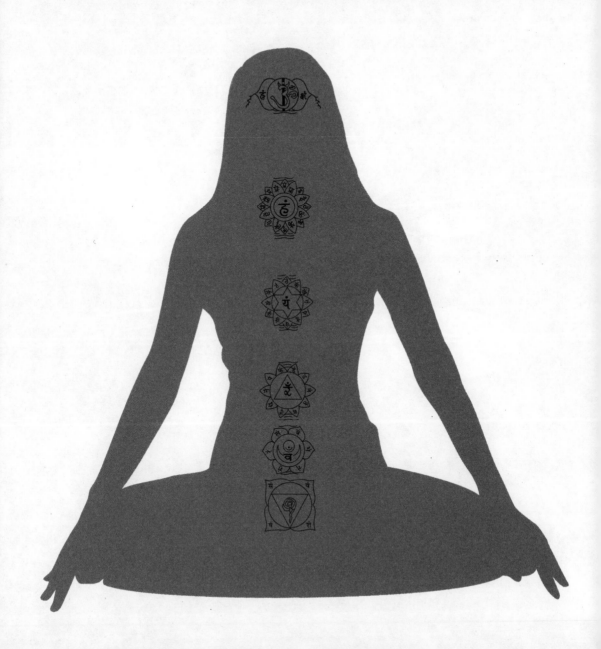

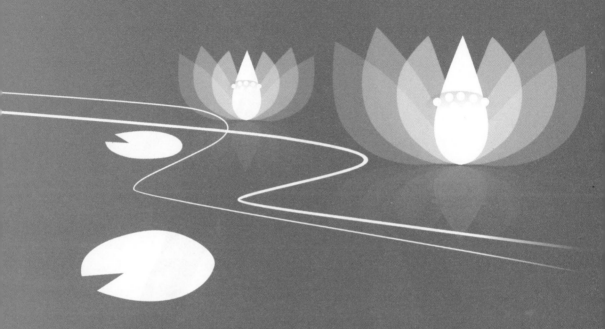

CHAPTER VII

YOGIC
DETOXIFICATION

Yogic Detoxification

Most ailments are the outcome of a toxic system. We ingest toxins from various sources – the foods we eat have many harmful chemicals as additives, preservatives, colourings and residue from pesticides and insecticides; the water we drink is treated with chemicals and the air we breathe is full of pollutants. It is the liver's job to detoxify the system, but when the toxins exceed in amount, its capacity to throw them out slows down and some of these harmful substances remain behind.

Furthermore, our body also produces waste continuously, which is meant to be removed by the eliminative system. But due to faulty eating habits and stress, this system becomes sluggish and the waste accumulates in the body. Inadequate evacuation of bowel becomes chronic, and the stale waste putrefies, leading to an environment acidic – a condition most suitable for fast multiplication of harmful microbes. These parasites produce still more toxins. Thus, the intestine becomes a storehouse of gas, acids and chemicals which get absorbed into the blood stream and are dumped into the body cells.

Tissues in the body are but individual entities, who act in a manner similar to human beings. They eat, drink, excrete, breathe, reproduce and die and understand each instruction of the brain and carry them out. They interact and empathise with each other to such an extent that if the tongue is enjoying the food, the cells of the stomach respond by working overtime to digest, no matter how heavy the food may be.

More than anything else, these cells want to live and function in a clean environment. The responsibility of doing the job well falls on the blood. If this fluid itself becomes impure, how can it remove the metabolic debris? The nourishment it carries also becomes toxic. Choked by toxins, the underfed tissues cannot function well, ushering in diseases. Sometimes the irritation caused to them makes them go wild and behave erratically and produce excessive cells. Cancer is the outcome.

This explains why most cancer patients have weak livers. They either had a weak liver to begin with, which could not detoxify the blood effectively, giving rise to the toxic condition of the body; or these people consumed far too much toxins for the liver to completely eliminate them. The extra work that this vital organ must have put in, has weakened it considerably.

The yogis of ancient India had understood that the body first needed to be cleansed to afford a cure for any ailment. Otherwise the energy generated through *asanas* and *pranayamas* would be used up to burn the toxic waste and there would not be enough energy to heal the system. Hence, they devised six cleansing techniques called *Shatkarma* out of which *Dhauti* (washing), especially, *Shankha Prakshyalana* is extremely important to cure cancer. Designed to clean the digestive tract, *Shankha Prakshyalana,* as the name suggests, accomplishes that task perfectly. The meaning of '*Shankha'* is a conch shell and '*Prakshyalana'* means washing. The digestive tract is as difficult to reach as the inside of a conch shell!

Shankha Prakshyalana is of two types:
1. *Guru Shankha Prakshyalana,* the major one and
2. *Laghoo Shankha Prakshyala,* the minor one.

It is the former that detoxifies the entire system in the shortest possible time. This practice involves drinking 20-30 glasses of saline water (which dissolves the mucous wherein toxins are trapped), practicing five *asanas* thereafter, and evacuating the bowel. First the intestine is emptied, and then, water circulating all over the body removes the toxins stored in the cells and flushes them out of the system. Thus in a few hours, the body is 'washed clean' and the blood is made pure.

Guru Shankha Prakshyalana, also, improves the digestive health. This practice empties the intestine completely and food is taken only after forty-five minutes. This means the entire digestive system including the liver have no digestive work to do in that interim time. This well-deserved rest does wonders to these body parts and they revive and become strong again. The now-strong liver gets on the job again of working the digestive system efficiently. It is essential to do *Guru Shankha Prakshyalana* under expert supervision, as it is a complicated process with many rules and regulations that must be followed to avoid undesirable consequences. In the absence of competent supervision, the minor version can be undertaken. This practice may not be as wonderful as the major one, but is safer and when practiced for five consecutive days in the beginning, it is effective enough for the purpose.

The old and infirm, heart patients or people with hernia or severe backache, must not attempt either of these practices on their own.

Laghoo Shankha Prakshyalana

- Have a light and early dinner the previous evening. In the morning, heat up 6 glasses of water.
- The temperature of the water should be such that though hot, you should be able to drink it quickly.
- Add 2 tea spoons of salt and mix well.

- According to texts, ½ tsp should be put in a glass of water, but you should start with less and increase later if necessary.

Drink 2 glasses of this saline water quickly and practice the following *asanas*:

Tadasana

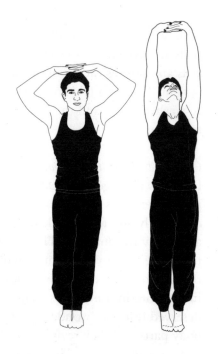

- Stand straight with feet together.
- Interlock the fingers and extend arms above the head.
- Turn the palms out.
- Inhaling, rise to your toes; stretch and turn your face up to look at the hands.
- Exhaling, bang your heels down while bringing the hands to the head and returning the face to the normal position.

Repeat 8 times.

Tiryaka Tadasana

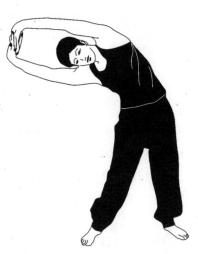

- Stand straight with legs apart.
- Interlock fingers and stretch your arms over the head with the palms facing up.
- Inhale.
- Exhaling, bend to your left from the waist.
- Inhaling, return to the upright position
- Exhaling, bend to the right.

- Inhaling, return.

Repeat 4 times.

Kati Chakrasana

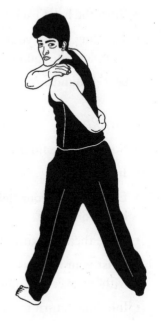

- Stand with legs apart and arms out on the side.
- Inhale.
- Exhaling, twist your body to the left from your waist and keep the right hand on your left shoulder. At the same time, take the left arm behind and keep the left hand on the right side of the waist with palm turned out.
- Inhaling, return to the starting position. Repeat on the other side to complete the round.

Practice 4 rounds.

Triyaka Bhujangasana

- Lie down on your stomach.
- Keep the hands flat on the ground and near the chest.
- Inhaling, turn your face up while stretching the neck. Rise fully.

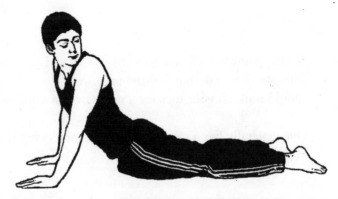

- Holding the breath in, turn your head over the left shoulder to look at your feet.
- Turn the head back to the front.
- Exhaling, lower yourself to the ground. Practice on the other side to complete the round.

Repeat 4 rounds.

Udarakh

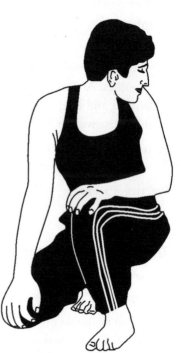

- Squat on the floor with hands on the knees.
- Inhale.
- Exhaling, lift your right heel and turn the body to the left.
- Place the right knee near the left foot.
- Twist your body as much as possible without over straining it.
- Inhaling, return to the starting position.
- Practice on the other side to complete the round.

Repeat 4 rounds.

At this point you should go to the toilet and defecate. If you do not feel the urge, you should walk on your toes for a while or just stroll but avoid sitting.

One generally has a clear motion after practicing the *Laghoo Shankha Prakshyalana*.

After cleansing the bowels, practice *Kunjal*.

TECHNIQUE:

- Heat up 2 glasses of water.
- Add 2-3 tsps salt and mix.
- Drink the water quickly
- Insert the first and second fingers of the right hand into your mouth.
- Press the tongue or touch its base.
- While pressing the stomach with the left hand.

The water will gush out.

Keep pressing the tongue intermittently to expel most of the water.

NOTE: Before attempting *Laghoo Shankha Prakshyalana*, you should be familiar with *Kunjal*. Unless you are able to bring out the water, do not practice *Laghoo Shankha Prakshyalana*; otherwise, there will be too much saline water in the body which may lead to *Gunu Shankha Prakshyalana*. In such a case, many rules and regulations have to be followed which you may not be able to handle.

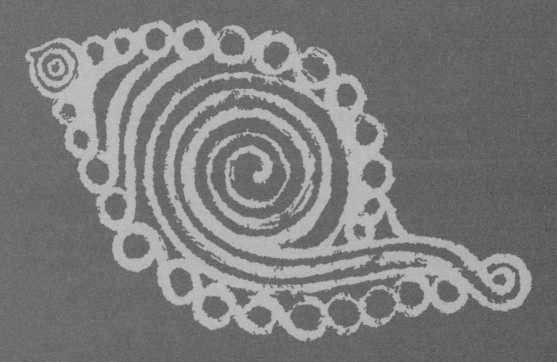

CHAPTER VIII

YOUR WILL
TO BE CURED

Your Will to be Cured

The power of one's will is unimaginable and history is its proof. Many a great men have exhibited it from time to time. That Napoleon could live continuously for four months on horseback during the first Italian campaign is no ordinary feat. Mughal Emperor Babar, who ruled India in the early sixth century amazed everyone with his extraordinary will when his son Humayun fell critically ill. In spite of all available treatments, the prince's condition continued to deteriorate and there was little hope for his recovery. The emperor, then, decided to save his son by using any means. He went around Humayun's bed three times with a strong resolution to trade off his life for his son's. From that day onwards, the prince started gaining health and recovered fully, while Babar fell ill and died. The emperor was only in his fifties, and was of strong built.

The power of will lies in the subconscious mind. If it has decided to cure a disease, nothing can stop it from doing so. In the past, epidemics of plague, cholera and yellow fever claimed millions of lives, but again, millions of lives were unaffected, despite being exposed to those deadly microbes. It is not because of any wonder drug, but because of their subconscious mind which decided to protect them by making the immune system produce the right anti-bodies to destroy the invaders. Furthermore, automatic regression of cancer is not an unknown phenomenon.

The subconscious, every second of the day, keeps a strict vigil over our body and protects it from all danger.

This is why we can sleep on a twelve inches wide bed and still not fall off. Protecting us from all ailments including cancer is a child's play for this mind.

Our body routinely produces cancerous cells, but the subconscious immediately detects it and mobilises the T cells to devour the freak ones. It is only when the subconscious does not bother that the cancerous cells are left to grow and claim one's life. This uncooperative attitude of the subconscious is mainly due to stress and once that is gotten rid of, the subconscious behaviour changes

The subconscious can be accessed and influenced only when the body and the conscious mind are completely relaxed – a state brought about by a yogic relaxation technique called *Yoga Nidra*. During this practice, the brain waves change from the usual beta to alpha, the waves generally produced during sleep or when the mind is completely inactive.

Yoga Nidra is highly therapeutic. It brings about optimum relaxation of the blood vessels leading to better blood flow to the body tissues. If the blood is pure, it results in better nourishment and proper oxygenation for the cells in the body and more efficient elimination of the metabolic waste.

With better blood flow to the tissues, the body parts are quickly and effectively rejuvenated. The relaxation during *Yoga Nidra* is such that, half an hour of it is known to have the same effect on the system as does two hours of deep sleep. Practised at bedtime, it not only removes all traces of stress from the body and mind, but also induces sound sleep.

Practicing it twice or thrice a day provides all the rest one needs to repair and rejuvenate one's system completely. Many mind control methods have similar techniques to relax the body. But *Yoga Nidra* follows a sequence matching the sequential pattern formed in the brain by the nerves of the corresponding body parts. This allows the mind to glide smoothly over the body without getting confused.

Though a live voice is most effective, recorded *Yoga Nidra* is more practical and has almost the same result. This practice can be done any time provided the stomach is not full. It can also be practiced in any position, though *Shavasana* is the best.

TECHNIQUE

(To be recorded and played)

- Lie down in *Shavasana* and close your eyes. Relax your body and make yourself comfortable. Make sure the clothes you are wearing are loose.

- Count 50 breaths backwards. Breathing should be absolutely spontaneous. Visualise your body for about 30 seconds. Make a resolution and repeat it 3 times sincerely in your mind.

- Now, let your mind wander over your body repeating the name of each part mentally, as is written below and visualise that part:

Right hand thumb—the tip—nail—first joint—second joint—index finger—tip—nail—first joint—second joint—third joint—middle finger—tip—nail—first joint—second joint—third joint—ring finger—tip—nail—first joint—second joint—third joint—palm—center of the palm—back of the hand—wrist—forearm—elbow—upper arm—shoulder—armpit—right side of the trunk—waist—right hip—right thigh—knee—calf—shin—ankle—heel—sole—top of the foot—the big toe—tip—nail—first joint—second joint—second toe—tip—nail—first joint—second joint—third joint—third toe—tip-nail—first joint—second joint—third joint—fourth toe—tip—nail—first joint—second joint—third joint—fifth toe—tip—nail—first joint—second joint—third joint.

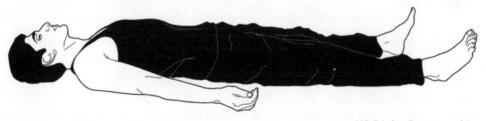

Left hand thumb – complete the left side in the same manner.

Right shoulder blade—left shoulder blade—right side of the back—left side of the back—spine—right hip—left hip—right heel—left heel—back of the neck—back of the head—top of the head—forehead—right eyebrow—left eyebrow—right eye—left eye—middle of the eyebrows—right temple—left temple—right ear—left ear—right cheek—left cheek—right nostril—left nostril—tip of the nose—upper lip—lower lip—both lips together—chin—jaw—neck—right collarbone—left collarbone—right side of the chest—left side of the chest—navel—abdomen.

Now take your mind into the body—teeth—tongue—throat—food pipe—windpipe— right lung—left lung—heart—liver—stomach—small intestine—large intestine—right kidney—left kidney—bladder—(add uterus and ovaries for ladies)—all the bones— all the blood vessels—the brain—and all the nerves—the whole body—the whole body—the whole body—the whole body—and the whole body.

Let your mind wander once or twice more over the body parts as described above.

Now you will visualise a few healing symbols—green meadow—snowy mountains—calm lake—white clouds—a mango tree—a white rose—torrential rain—blue sky—birds in flight—sandy bank of a wide river—a sea with massive waves—the expanding beach—starlit night—full moon—and a steady candle flame.

Visualise your heart—visualise a tiny being sitting in it and smiling at you—its eyes are full of love for you—you smile back and send lots of love to it too—you are feeling very happy.

Remember your resolution and repeat it thrice in your mind. Be aware of your body—be aware of the room you are in—move your body—stretch it—and slowly open your eyes.

The practice of *Yoga Nidra* is over.

Prana Vidya

This technique, done after *Yoga Nidra,* makes the latter even more potent. It involves visualising *prana* and healing various parts of the body with it. The traditional *Prana Vidya* is said to cure all diseases, even without the support of any other treatment. But that calls for absolute precision and a high degree of concentration, because, as it involves drawing *prana* from the *kundalini*, it can lead to unwanted consequences if mishandled. That is why many prefer to use the simplified version, which does not disturb the *kundalini*. Instead, it uses the external *prana* that can do no harm even if improperly practiced. *Prana Vidya* can be added in the end of *Yoga Nidra* or practiced separately.

TECHNIQUE

Keep your body relaxed and immobile and the eyes closed. Count your breaths backward from 100 to 1.

Imagine the room you are in is filled with golden light, and when you inhale, your body expands and soaks in that energy through every pore. When you breath out, imagine dirty air is coming out of your nose. After about five minutes, imagine the exhaled air gradually turning colourless. Feel your body tingling with an abundance of the life force. Visualise your physician pronouncing that your disease is cured and congratulating you. Visualise you telling everybody how you have cured yourself. They all are very happy, so are you. Bring a smile to your face and slowly open your eyes.

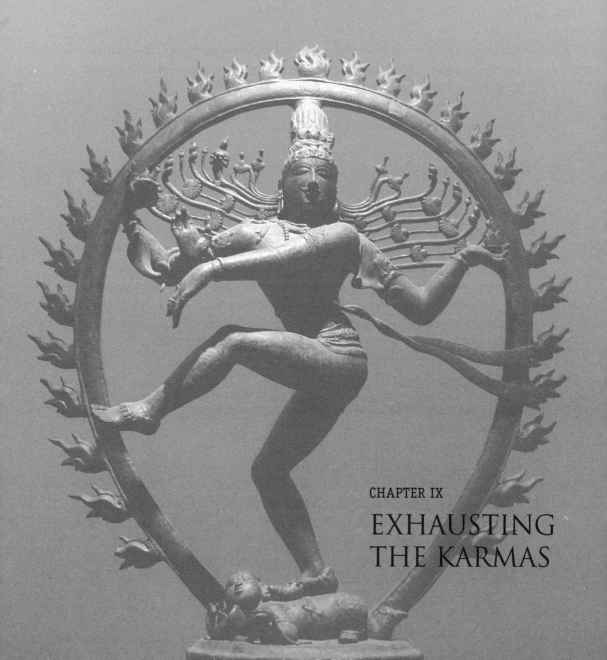

CHAPTER IX

EXHAUSTING
THE KARMAS

Exhausting the Karmas

In this world, everything follows the laws of cause and effect. Innumerable thoughts plague our minds every moment of the day and leave without making any impact only to be forgotten. However, there are some thoughts that make us reflect upon them again and again. They are known as *vrittis*, loosely meaning idea. These ideas make grooves in the subconscious and remain there permanently. When a group of similar ideas accumulate, it becomes a belief. Such a belief is known as a *sanskara* or archetype, which affects every aspect of our personality – our nature, character, reflexes and response. These elements become the cause for our actions, which in turn become the cause for yet another set of actions, and in this manner, an unbroken chain of cause and effect is created that controls our lives and thus the sum total of our *samskaras* is called our *karma* or destiny.

According to yoga, *samskaras* accumulate from the moment we enter our mother's womb. It is said that the day the soul enters the body of a foetus (believed to happen in the fourth month of pregnancy) every thought of the mother, and after birth, every experience of the baby is recorded by the subconscious.

Indian philosophy goes back in time and says that *samskara* is not acquired in this life alone, but carried forward from all our previous births.

According to it, when a person dies, the subtle body along with the stored archetypes, leaves the gross body of flesh and bones and based on its *karma*, finds a suitable new body and a new environment to enjoy or suffer the consequences, as the case may be.

Whether or not one believes in the concept of transmigration, our negative thoughts of this life are enough to create trouble for us. With excessive negative *samskaras*, the subconscious may become so negative that it may not believe in the conscious mind's positive resolution and reject it altogether. Hence, to afford a cure, the negative archetypes need to be first removed from the mind. *Samskaras* cannot be wished away nor ended automatically; they can be either transferred or worked upon. Often people heal others by their thoughts or techniques. Unknowingly, they might be transferring the patient's *karma* onto themselves. It is said that many great souls have done that on their own accord.

Ramakrishna Parmahamsa who is known to have given relief to any number of sufferers, developed throat cancer, perhaps, because he took the negative *karma* of those people onto himself.

Karmas should be ideally exhausted by one's own effort and the masters of the ancient world have recommended various methods to achieve that. Some of them are:

- *Mauna*: observation of silence
- *Mantra*
- *Tapasya*: austerity
- Prayer
- *Bhajan and kirtan*: devotional songs
- Meditation

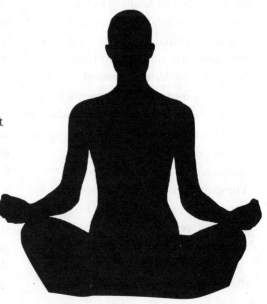

Meditation not only purges the stored negative archetypes, but also de-stresses the mind completely. As stress is one of the major causes of cancer, meditation goes a long way in alleviating the disease. During meditation, profound changes occur in the body to indicate its highly relaxed state. The heartbeat and respiration become slow, the brain waves change from beta to alpha and theta and lactic acid, the stress hormone, is eliminated three times faster during this practice than during normal sleep.

Of all the forms of meditation, *antar mauna* is extremely effective to purge the stored negative thoughts. The *vrittis* or archetypes are brought out of the inner recesses of the mind. We see them in the forms they are stored – colours, symbols and figures. When they are confronted by the conscious mind, they are automatically released. Once that happens, the positive resolution to get well becomes doubly effective.

MEDITATION
Sit in one of the following meditative postures:

Padmasana

- Sit on the floor and cross your legs.
- Put the right foot on the left thigh.
- Put the left foot on the right thigh.

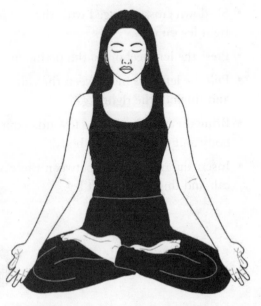

Ardha Padmasana

- Sit down on the floor.
- Put the right foot on the left thigh or the left foot on the right thigh.
- The other leg remains as it is.

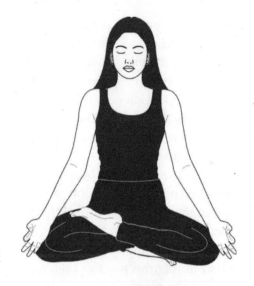

Siddhaasana

Siddhaasana guards prostate health and helps prevent prostate cancer.

- Sit down crossed-legged with the right leg on top.
- Press the left heel on to the perineum.
- Pull the left toes in between the calf and thigh of the right leg.
- Bring the right heel close towards your body and press it on the body.
- Insert the right toes in between the calf and thigh of the left leg.

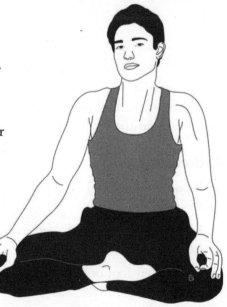

Sukhasana

Sit down and simply cross your legs.

Whichever *asana* you choose for meditation, you should be able to sit in that position without moving the body for at least twenty minutes. Movement during this practice can disrupt the energy flow and negate the effect of meditation. If your body is too stiff to assume any of the above mentioned *asanas*, you can do it in *Shavasana*. But in this *asana* the chances of dozing off to sleep are very high and that too can negate the effect of meditation. So, if you meditate in *Shavasana*, you have to be extra careful to stay awake all through the practice. You should keep suggesting to yourself every now and then that you have to remain alert till the end.

- Assume the posture of your choice.
- Straighten your body.
- Make your body still.
- Concentrate on your body.
- Concentrate on the stillness of your body.
- Visualise your body from the front for 10 to 15 seconds.
- Visualise it from the right side for 10 to 15 seconds; do the same from the back and then from the left, and again from the front.
- Release tension from each part of your body one by one as follows:
  - Think of your forehead ... eyebrows ... (do not frown) eyes ... relax the eyelids by shutting them very gently.
  - Now think of your lips ... as if they are about to part.
  - Come down towards the jaw ... unclench the teeth and drop the jaw.
  - Relax the shoulder.

- Do *gyan* or *Chin Mudra* and keep hands on the knees.
- Relax the legs.
- Concentrate on your breath.
- Let your breathing be spontaneous. Count your breaths backward from 100.
- After 100 breaths, set your mind free, but be watchful.
- Let thoughts come into your mind spontaneously and leave on their own.
- Do not interfere with your natural thinking process.
- Take note of each thought without getting involved; just be a dispassionate witness.
- After around 5 minutes, try to stop thinking and keep the mind blank for a minute or so. Now choose your thoughts, 1 at a time. Mull over 1 thought, discard it, bring another, think about it; discard it and bring yet another thought.
- Again, after around 5 minutes try and make your mind blank for a little

while. Visualize a candle flame in between your eyebrows and concentrate on it for 3-4 minutes.

- Before ending the session, chant '*Oum*' 7 times.

- For '*Oum*' chanting, first take a deep breath, and as you exhale say a long 'O'; after that chant a short 'U' and again follow it with a long 'M' till your lungs are empty.

- Repeat this process.

- Be aware of your body.

- Be aware of the external sounds. Slowly open your eyes.

CAUTION: Do not continue practicing meditation if the legs have become numb. If that happens every time you meditate, you may try with another meditative posture.

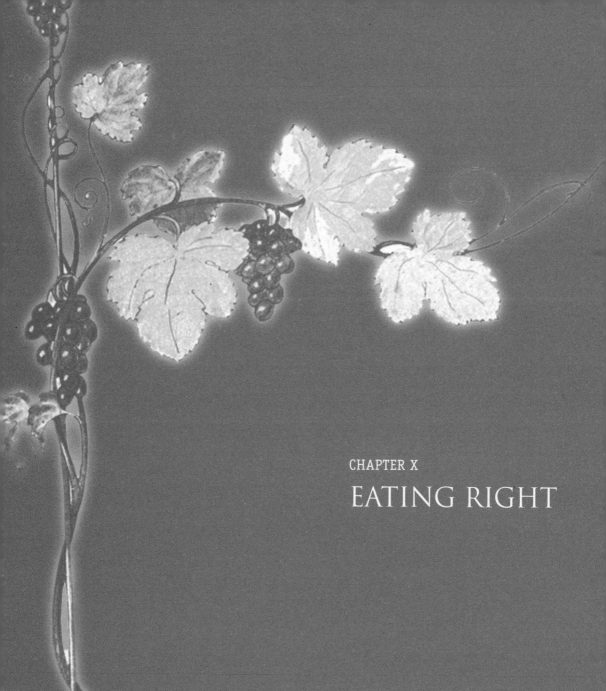

CHAPTER X
EATING RIGHT

Eating Right

Food plays a very important role in curing cancer, as wrong food can negate the effect of any treatment including yoga. A foodstuff should not be taken just because it is rich in specific nutrients or is supposed to have certain therapeutic qualities, as no food item is universally good or bad. It is one's body system that determines whether an item is beneficial or harmful. For instance, orange might be an excellent fruit, but for an arthritis patient, it can immediately aggravate the pain. If the person continues to have this fruit, then no therapy, no matter how effective, can cure the disease. Hence, utmost importance should be given on our choice of food.

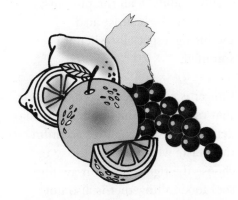

As cancer cells seem to thrive in an acidic medium and die within three hours when kept in an alkaline solution, all acid and acid-forming foods should be strictly avoided. Sour tasting food such as lemon, vinegar are acidic, while all proteins such as meat, chicken, fish, eggs, peanuts, cashew nuts, beans, black gram are acid forming – uric acid being the end product in protein metabolism. Also, proteins need hydrochloric acid to be digested – which means the more the protein, the more acidic the body becomes.

Making the food predominantly alkaline is the only way to negate the adverse effects of this unavoidable nutrient. Most fruits and vegetables are alkaline in nature, so are raw vegetables and cereals, while cooked food with spices such as red chilies, is highly acidic. Of all the proteins, green gram is the least acid producing, especially when it is sprouted.

Cancer is considered a cold disease that calls for heating food. Ayurveda determines food qualities according to their taste which makes it easy to choose the right ones. But avoiding cool foods alltogether is also not reccommended – they should be included in smaller quantity in the proportion relevant to the disease. Food classification according to *Ayurveda*:

- Sweet: cold and moisture producing
- Saline: warm, bitter dry and cool
- Sour: cool
- Pungent: warm
- Astringent: heavy and cool

To further increase the temperature of the essential cooling food, some heat-inducing spices such as saffron, nutmeg, ginger, garlic, turmeric and mace should be used.

In the daily diet of a cancer patient, some extremely therapeutic foods should be included. Simultaneously, care should be taken to consume all the nutrients, as nutritional deficiency is a cause of cancer as well. In 1950, a doctor observed that all his cancer patients were severely deficient in calcium and when he treated them with this mineral, each terminal case survived. Calcium is anti-cancerous because it is essential for phagocyte cells to attach and ingest cancer causing foreign matter.

Deficiency of these nutrients can also cause cancer:

- **Iron:** this mineral is essential for the production of anti-bodies and enzymes made by the immune cells.
- **Zinc:** thymus, the master gland of the immune system shrinks with inadequate zinc leading to a weak immune system.

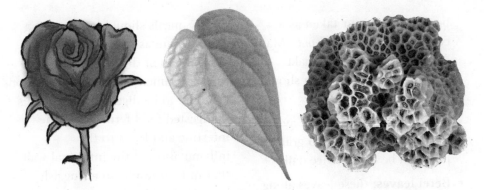

- **Magnesium:** the combination of calcium and magnesium is essential for antibody production.

- **Selenium and Vitamin E:** there is no antibody without these two nutrients.

- **Vitamin A and C:** These are the main food for the immune cells.

- **B-Complex:** a baby's thymus gland is larger and the immune system stronger if the mother has had a good supply of this vitamin.

These food items are extremely therapeutic for this ailment and must be taken regularly:

- **Turmeric:** is a powerful anti-oxidant and also anti-cancerous

- Garlic eaters have the lowest incidence of cancer

Coral: neutralises body acid

- **Aloevera:** a strong immunity booster

- Yellow fruits and vegetables are powerful anti-oxidants

- **Basil:** these natural Vitamin A rich leaves, fights cancer by maintaining a healthy thymus

- **Mushroom:** is a rich source of zinc, the nutrient necessary to produce enzymes needed for elimination of routinely produced cancer cells

- **Wheat grass juice:** in the treatment of cancer, its therapeutic value has been made well known by Anna Wigmore

- **Rose:** rosehips are the richest source of vitamin C and hence a very powerful antioxidant. It can be taken as it is or taken as a confection callled 'gulkand'. Many Ayurvedic pharmacies make gulkand with coral, which should be taken regularly

- **Aloevera:** bottled juice is available in the market. About 25 grams of juice can be taken twice daily
- **Betel leaves:** these leaves along with coconut and nutmeg are known to regress cancerous growth, especially in the mouth.

In India, betel is generally taken after meals. Condiments such as clove, mace, nutmeg, fennel seeds, omum, green cardamom and coriander seeds are put in the betel leaf along with betel nut. It is then rolled into a neat packet and chewed as all the ingredients used in the betel are powerful digestives. Furthermore, the chewing itself brings about copious amounts of saliva that helps in digestion, but the saliva itself is a strong antacid. Alternatively, the juice of one leaf can be taken with honey twice daily.

How to eat is as important as what to eat for better utilsation of food.

Firstly, meals should be taken in a relaxed state as stress leads to suppression of digestive juices and food consumed under such conditions is bound to be digested poorly. This undigested food ferments in the intestine and leads to the inflammation of the intestinal wall that in turn results in a sluggish intestine and inadequate evacuation. Therefore, the system should be de-stressed before meals for which the following techniques are quick and effective.

OUM CHANTING
ABDOMINAL BREATHING.
MENTAL ANULOME-VILOMA

Oum chanting: it has been seen that when Oum is pronounced, the brain immedietely produces alpha waves indicating a relaxed state. If chanting aloud is not possible, thinking of the sound also helps.

ABDOMINAL BREATHING
(10 times):

First, breathe in to fill up the the lower part of the lungs; breathe more to fill up the chest and then deeper to lift the shoulder up. To exhale, first, release the air from the top, then the middle and lastly from the lowest part.

MENTAL ANULOMA-VILOMA
(1-2 minutes)

For this you only need to imagine that you are breathing in from the left nostril and breathing out from the right and then breathing in from the right and breathing out from the left.

Secondly, food should be taken when the *Pingala Nadi* is active. This indicates that the left hemisphere responsible for physical activities such as digestion and elimination is at its best. We eat food when the body is not prepared to process it. If one is eating during the *Ida Nadi* phase, that is, when the right hemisphere of the brain, which controls mental activities is active, food taken at that time is bound to be poorly digested.

Therefore, check the flow of breath before a meal. If the left is flowing, wait for it to change naturally, which normally takes about an hour or do the following simple yogic practice to change it.

- Kneel down and sit on your feet, placing the hands under the opposite armpits

- Maintain the posture for 2 to 3 minutes

- Remove the left hand from the right armpit and check the flow. Continue the *asana* for some more time if the flow hasn't changed.

Thirdly, avoid eating in the standing position as gravity pulls the blood down to the legs, whereas the blood should concentrate around the stomach for better digestion. For that matter, sitting in the cross leg posture is the ideal position for eating. Yoga recommends

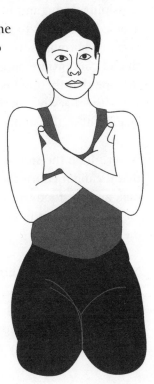

sitting in *Vajarasana* for 10-20 minutes after meals. In this position, the blood is squeezed up from the legs to pool near the stomach.

Yoga also recommends eating with hands and not with forks and spoons as the *prana* coming out of the fingers not only energises the food, but also gets re-absorbed into the system.

Gossiping during meals should be avoided as it leads to the secretion of negative hormones. Instead, one should concentrate on the food and imagine that the food is being fed to *agni* – the digestive fire supposed to be present in the stomach.

Never fill up the stomach so much that it cannot churn the contents well, and the food will remain there for a long time and draw more acid in the process.

Needless to say, you should chew your food well. Not only does this help in making the food go easy on the stomach, but mastication draws more saliva which is a highly alkaline

substance that neutralises the acidic food in the stomach.

Lastly, avoid using the microwave to cook or even to reheat. If food is heated or cooked in a microwave, the vitamins may remain intact, but the *prana* will be completely destroyed.

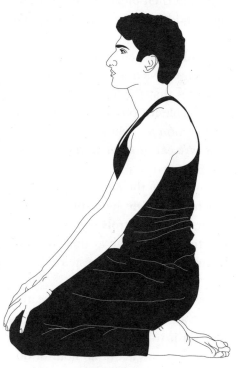

Vajrasana

It is said that repeating the following
mantra ensures perfect digestion.

Agastyam Kumbhakaranam cha
Shameencha Vaada Vaanalam
Bhojanam Pachanaarthaaye
Smaredabhyamcha Panchakam

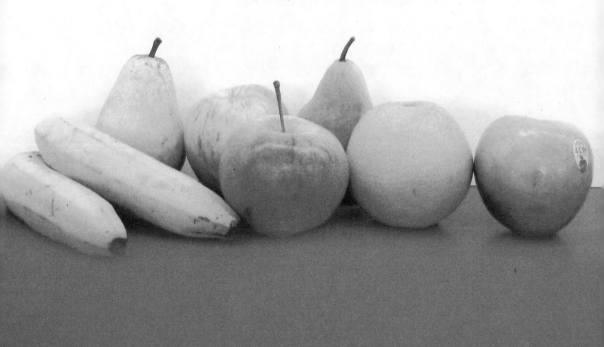

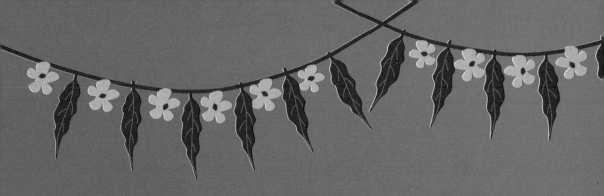

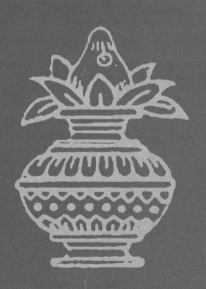

CHAPTER XI

IMPORTANT
ADDITIONS

Important Additions

The treatment for cancer should be as expansive as possible to contain the disease at the earliest. One of the most effective treatments is urine therapy or *Amroli*, which I have recommended to all my cancer patients and this has had extremely wonderful results.

AMROLI

An ancient *tantric* practice of India meant to maintain perfect health, *Amroli*, is the yogic term for urine therapy, which literally means the way to immortality. Scriptures written five thousand years ago say that by drinking urine every morning, all diseases in the body caused by *'vata'* (gas) *'pitta'* (acid) and *'kapha'* (mucus) are destroyed; digestion is improved and the body becomes strong. It is believed that the body produces urine appropriate to cure the illnesses of that time.

Urine's effect on cancer has been remarkable. Research on the components of urine has yielded extremely positive results as seen from the following:

- H 11 stops the growth of cancer cells and decreases cancerous growth.

- Directin brings discipline into the wild cancer cells by aligning them in a straight line.

- Isolated from urine by Nobel Laureate Albert S. Gyorgi, Methyle glyoxal destroys cancer cells.

- A steroid called DHEA seems to cure cancer.

Urine is a natural healer, known to heal wounds and kill microbes effectively. It can give relief from an infected toothache in minutes. A healthy person's urine is sterile and contains no bacteria, as it prevents germs from breeding and growing. The right diet during *Amaroli* should be devoid of non-vegetarian foods, onions and garlic and kept low in proteins, acids, salt, milk and its products, fruits, pulses and alcohol. Simply cooked rice, whole wheat bread and vegetables are the safest food. This leads to urine being odourless and taste mild.

The first flow is meant to clear out the urethra, while the last flow contains nothing valuable and so only the mid-stream urine should be used. For a cure, it should be taken 3 times a day – the first thing in the morning, 1 hour after lunch and 1 hour after dinner. As a preventive, the morning flow, alone, is sufficient. It is necessary to drink 8-10 glasses of water everyday to keep the urine diluted. 1 or 2 days of urine fast is also an excellent way to detoxify and rejuvenate the system. This is also an effective alternative to *Guru Shankha Prakshyalana*. Nothing, but urine and water, should be taken.

Initially, one may experience some problems such as vomiting, loose motions, skin eruptions, mild fever and cold and cough. These are mere symptoms of toxins being purged, and passed off in a few days*.

FASTING

Fasting for inner purification is an age old practice in many religions. Traditional Hindus fast at least twice a month, mostly on the eleventh day of the moon. Though it has acquired a religious flavour, fasting is anything but that. It is woven into a religion only to encourage people to practice it sincerely and acquire its beneficial effects.

The benefits of a fast are many. First,

*NOTE: People with liver, kidney and heart diseases should not attempt this therapy. Also, it should not be commenced while one is under any medication. It can be taken up after at least a week of discontinuing the medicine. People with pus filled urine and those who do not want to use their own urine can take that of a cow. Now a day, many organisations are marketing sterile bottled cow urine and even in tablet form, for this purpose.

when there is no digestion to be done, the digestive organs, including the liver, get a chance to rest and rejuvenate. Secondly, the energy saved from digestion, is diverted for elimination of body toxins. Since in cancer, a toxic body is a major hindrance to cure, fasting becomes helpful; and lastly, the body destroys its weak and old tissues that unnecessarily consume its reserve energy. Looking after fewer cells helps it to live longer. Dr. Roy Walford reported to have doubled the life span of some mice by withdrawing their food for two days a week.

Some therapies such as Naturopathy, recommend long fasts with complete rest to let the body rectify the inherent defects in its own way. Such fasts need to be monitored scientifically to prevent harm to the system. But short fasts, of 1 or 2 days duration, 2-3 times a month, can be done on one's own for an effective aid to cure cancer.

PRAYER

Sometime back a miraculous case was reported from an established hospital in the U.S. The family members of a cancer patient, on his death bed, had gathered round him to pray for his recovery, as the doctors had predicted a lifespan of less than a week for him. Days rolled by, and he regained his health and soon his cancer was gone. Another interesting reported case is that of T. Suji of Japan. He, too, according to his doctor, had a few days to live. He prayed for around seventeen hours a day. A few days later, he vomited blood, which when tested, had no cancer cells, and surprisingly, it contained a substance with anti-cancerous properties. Later, the serum was taken from his blood to treat other cancer patients. So pray if you have faith. You can also do prayer breathing which has helped many of my cancer patients. For this you have to inhale 7 counts while mentally chanting:

O God please make me perfectly healthy
1   2   3   4   5   6   7

Hold your breath for 1 count and say '*Oum*' mentally. Then exhale for 7 counts, saying the same sentence.

Again hold your breath for 1 count, and repeat '*Oum*' mentally.

Repeat for 5-10 minutes or more, as many times during the day as you can.

BHAJAN KIRTAN

These are devotional music. While the former is a poem, the latter involves singing 1 or 2 sentences, bearing the lord's names repeatedly. Both generally involve groups where everybody participates vocally and give beats with various instruments or by simply clapping.

Bhajan-kirtan belong to *Nada* Yoga – the yoga of sound. According to this yoga, the seven musical notes correspond to the seven major *chakras* or energy centers located on the spinal chord, near the nerve plexi. The resonance of a particular note stimulates the corresponding *chakra* into action, which in turn activates the area around it, especially the closest nerve plexus, stabilising the functions of the glands and organs connected to it.

There are other advantages of *bhajan* and *kirtan*. First, music automatically attracts the mind and holds it captive, not allowing it to brood over negative disease causing thoughts. This in turn facilitates healing. Broadly speaking, *kirtans* are based on the names of deities, which are, in fact, *mantras*. Secondly, when done for 20 minutes continuously, the rhythmic beating of musical instruments have been scientifically proven to be extremely de-stressing. The instruments used for *bhajan* and *kirtan* like *mridangam* and *manjira* themselves, have a deep and positive effect on our body and psyche. In *Nada yoga* meditation, where the mind is made to go within and explore the inner sounds, one does hear the sounds of these instruments as the mind becomes more and more sensitive; and lastly *bhajan* and *kirtan* involve devotion which itself is a powerful healer.

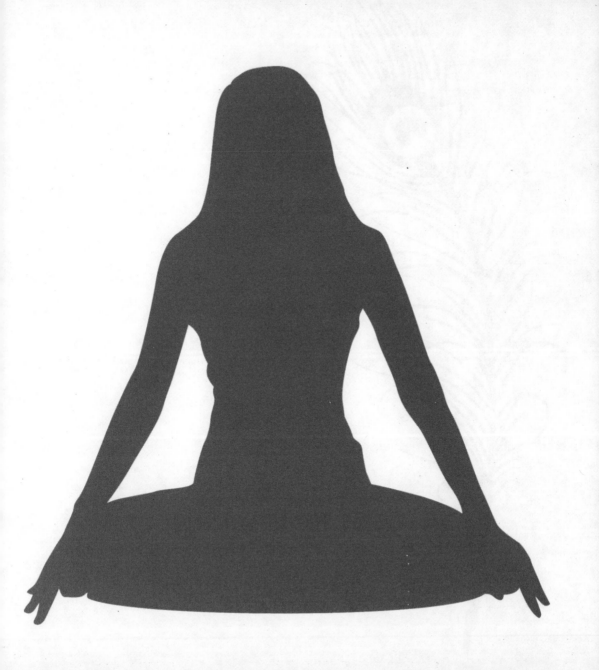

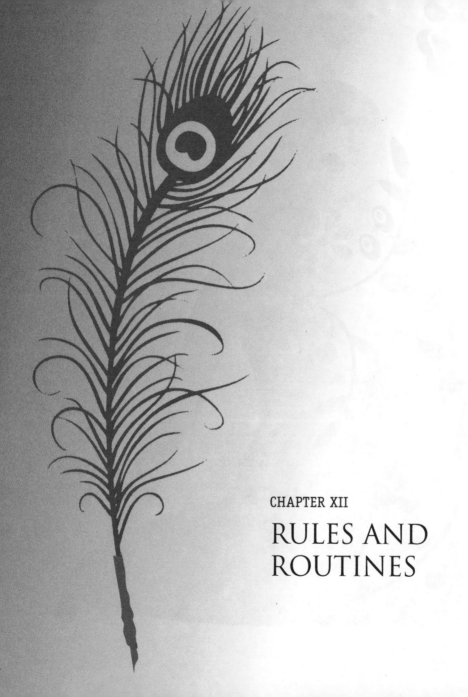

CHAPTER XII

RULES AND ROUTINES

Rules and Routines

Like every other system, yoga too has certain rules, which must be followed to avoid unpleasant consequences.

- *Yogaasanas* must be done on an empty stomach. This is because *asanas* work by drawing blood to a target area for healing. Since the amount of blood is constant in the body, this task is accomplished by taking the fluid away from the other body parts. After a meal, the stomach needs more blood for proper digestion and taking it away from this organ, can affect the digestion adversely. In the long run, this can damage the digestive system.

- Even meditation and *Yoga Nidra* done after meals can be harmful. These practices bring the inner body temperature down, whereas for good digestion, adequate body heat is essential. As mentioned earlier, undigested food is a major source of ailments. That is why yoga is ideally practiced in the morning before breakfast. One may also practice it 2-3 hours after a meal. *Pranayamas* should be done at least 4 hours after a meal.

- Loose cotton clothes should be worn during yoga practice, as the skin is unable to breathe well in synthetic ones. Woollens can be worn in cold weather.

- Yoga should be practiced in a well-ventilated, but not, windy room. A sudden drop in temperature can cause illness.

- Always maintain a straight back. The brain is connected with all the organs via the spine and any abnormal position of the spine can disturb the nerve current carrying messages to and from the brain.

- Practice yoga on a folded blanket. The back muscles, whose main concern is to support the spine, do not relax unless they are sure of the support from beneath, which they feel is inadequate on a soft spongy surface.

- Take food 10-15 minutes after completing a yoga routine, as the practice activates the glands and organs in the body. Also, the digestive juices start to pour into the stomach, which can harm its lining, if there is no food.

- Stick to the recommended number and duration of each *asana*. These practices work by shunting blood from one area to the other, which means that some body parts do not receive their usual quota of blood for a certain length of time. An important organ can withstand only a certain duration of deprivation without coming to any harm. The ancient yogis, with their profound insight and knowledge of the workings of the body, had fixed all the rules.

- *Shavasana* is recommended after each advanced *asana*, and should be followed strictly. This ensures proper blood flow to all the body tissues before pulling the blood away to a target area.

- Refrain from practicing yoga, if you have fever. During illness, the body's energy concentrates on rectifying the immediate problem and disturbing it during this time is unadvisable.

- Women should not practice yoga during the first 4 days of their monthly cycle.

- Practice yoga in semi darkness as the nerves automatically relax in this condition.

- Discontinue practice if you experience pain.

INTENSIVE YOGIC PROGRAMME FOR CANCER
(1 month)

6 a.m.

Laghu Shankha Prakshyalana –
5 consequitive days with salt;
thereafter once a week adding salt on
alternate weeks.

If your health does not permit the use
of so much salt, add it only on the
first day and then once in a fortnight.
If even that is not possible practice
Laghu Shankha Prakshyalana without
salt everyday for a month or so.

6.30 a.m.

Kunjal for a month and then twice a
week for 3 months; thereafter, once a
week for another 3 months.
(These 2 practices are essential in the
yogic treatment for cancer because as
long as there are toxins in the body, a
cure may not be possible.
Alternatively, you can try urine fast or
prolonged water and juice fast under
expert supervision.)

Bathe after *Kunjal*.

7.00 a.m.

Gayatri Mantra/Yagnya
A simpler alternative.

Listen to the recorded *mantra* and try
to follow it mentally.

Another alternative:
Write the *mantra* 'Ram' for
20-30 minutes.
or
do prayer breathing.

8.00 a.m.

Breakfast

11.00 a.m.

Yogic routine:

Oum chanting (7 times)

Leg rotation

Cycling

Utthan Padasana

Naukasana

Shavasana (10 breaths)

Surya Namaskar

Shavasana (10 breaths per round of *Surya Namaskar*)

Bhujangasana

Shalabhasana

Dhanurasana

Shavasana (10 breaths)

Shashankasana

Kandhrasana

Shavasana (10 breaths)

Paschimottanasana

Ardhamatsyendrasana

Shavasana (10 breaths)

Nadisodana Pranayama

Bhastika

Suryabheda

Yoni Mudra

Jalandhara Bandha

Uddiyana Bandha

Moola Bandha

Maha Bandha

Those who cannot practice the initial strenous *asanas*, up to *Surya Namaskar*, can substitute them with the simple *Pawan Muktasana* series. (See *Yoga for Busy People* by the same author)

Trataka
Chakra Shuddhi meditation
(not to be done for more than 1 month)

1.00 p.m.

Lunch

4.00 p.m.

Meditation and *Yoga Nidra*

5.00 p.m.

Juice

6.00 p.m.

Mahamrityunjaya Mantra/yagnya

Alternatively, listen to a recorded one or pay a priest to do it for you.

7.00 p.m.

Dinner

7.45 pm.

Group *kirtan* where you can participate is most affective. Else, sing along a recorded version.

8.15 p.m.

Dhanwantari Mantra. You can chant it or follow the recorded *mantra*.

Chant '*Oum*' 7 times before sleep.

To prevent the mind from thinking too much about the disease, fill in the rest of the time with *karmayoga* (the yoga of selfless physical labour) like gardening, stringing beads or flowers etc; yogic practices to improve other body parts such as the eyes, hair, gums etc; (see *Yoga and Meditation for All Ages* by the same author), massage, walking, and reading funny clean jokes that will induce laughter.

After a month, if tests show remarkable improvement, the *yagyas* and the former two *mantras* can be discontinued. *Suryabheda Pranayama* should dropped after the disease is cured. The body will not need so much heat afterwards.

Raw food recipes

This chapter contains recipes based on raw food essential to cure cancer. Those who cannot digest the food, may combine it with simply cooked food, but it should be kept as minimum as possible. They should focus more on fruits.

For the best result use organic food, and for salt use either sea salt or rock salt (the pinkish white one that is *Sendha namak* in Hindi).

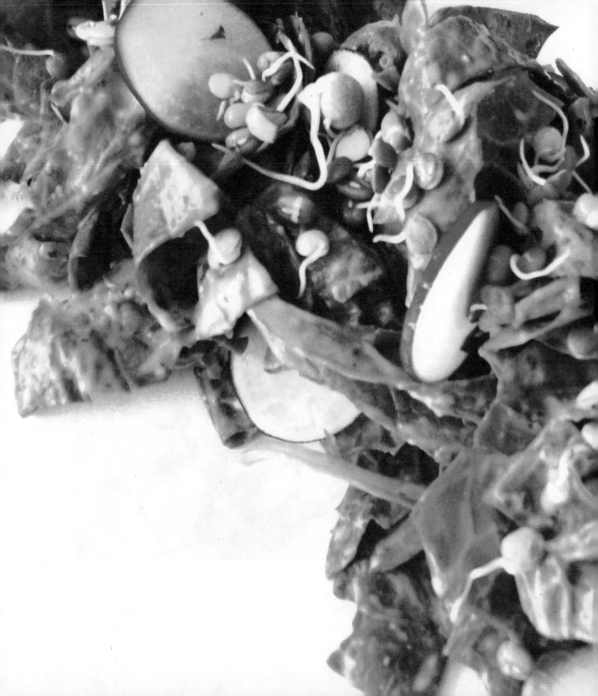

Apple-Blueberry Salad

Serves: 2   **Preparation time: 5 minutes**

Ingredients

4	ounces	blueberries
1	small	apple — diced small
2	tablespoons	currants
1	teaspoon	ginger — minced
1	tablespoon	apple juice
1	pinch	cinnamon
½	teaspoon	molasses
2	tablespoons	coconut meat, fresh

Apples are cleansing, especially to the liver and gall ballder, and they stimulate the appetite. They also help balance blood sugar, reduce cholesterol, ama, heavy metals and radiation from the body.

Blueberries also help balance blood sugar and cleanse the system.

Preparation method
Combine all ingredients and toss well.

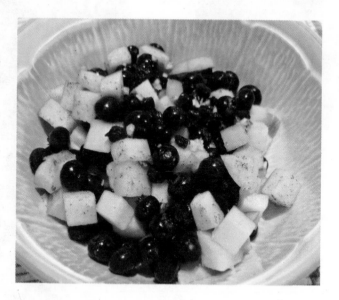

Per Serving (excluding unknown items): 127 Calories; 2g Fat (14.4% calories from fat); 1g Protein; 29g Carbohydrate; 5g Dietary Fibre; 0mg Cholesterol; 6mg Sodium. Exchanges: 0 Grain (Starch); 1½ Fruit; ½ Fat; 0 Other Carbohydrates.

Avocado Coconut Pudding

Serves: 5   **Preparation time: 10 minutes**

Ingredients

1		whole avocado
½	cup	coconut meat — from 1 fresh coconut
1¼	cups	coconut water — from 1 fresh coconut
2	tablespoons	lime juice — from 1 whole lime
5	tablespoons	honey — local and raw
3	pieces	mint sprigs

Coconut is cooling, soothing and nutritious to the body. It is beneficial to the lungs and skin and helps the body recuperate from infectious diseases.

Honey is Sattvic. It nourishes the whole body and helps increase immunity. When fresh, it is full of enzymes and minerals.

Preparation method
Place all in blender.

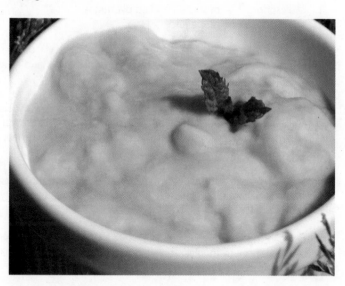

Per Serving (excluding unknown items): 171 Calories; 9g Fat (43.6% calories from fat); 2g Protein; 24g Carbohydrate; 2g Dietary Fibre; 0mg Cholesterol; 7mg Sodium. Exchanges: 0 Vegetable; ½ Fruit; 1½ Fat; 1 Other Carbohydrates.

Banana, Carrot and Fig Salad with Raisins and Alfalfa Sprouts

Serves: 2   **Preparation time: 5 minutes**

Ingredients

1	cup	alfalfa sprouts — 1 cup is around 2 ounces
1	whole	carrot — grated
1	whole	banana — sliced
2	whole	figs — fresh or dried, if dried soak overnight, sliced
1	tablespoon	raisins — soaked overnight
2	tablespoons	grape juice
2	pinches	salt

Alfalfa Sprouts are very cooling. They are highly nutritious and cleanse the blood and lymph.

Bananas are the most tonic fruits and help strengthen the body. They are high in minerals and can be used for hypertension and sugar or alcohol withdrawal. When ripe, they are a laxative; when unripe, they are useful in treating coughs, diarrhea, dysentery and hemorrhoids.

Carrots are cleansing and mildly tonic vegetables. High in nutrients, anti-oxidants and anti-carcinogens, they are effective in treating acne, diarrhea, dysentery, indigestion, liver, lung and skin disorders.

Figs are cleansing and tonic fruits. They balance acidity due to their alkalinity and are especially beneficial to the liver, gallbladder and urinary tract. A mild laxative, they help remove Ama from the body.

Preparation method

Place sprouts on a plate, spread out so that it acts as the base of the salad. Top with layers of grated carrots, then banana, figs and raisins. Drizzle lemon juice over the salad and sprinkle salt on top.

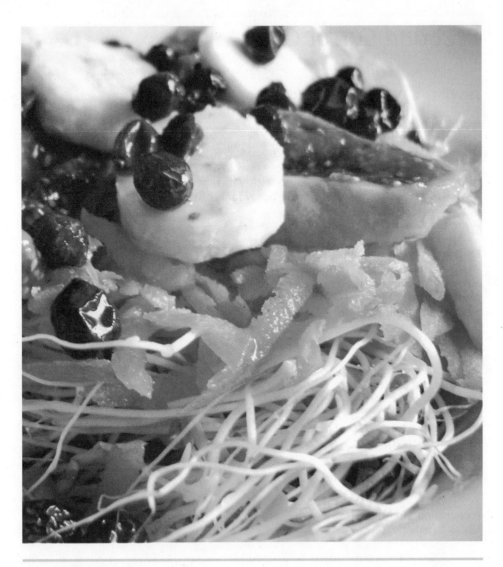

Per Serving (excluding unknown items): 135 Calories; 1g Fat (3.8% calories from fat); 2g Protein; 34g Carbohydrate; 5g Dietary Fibre; 0mg Cholesterol; 149mg Sodium. Exchanges: 0 Lean Meat; 1 Vegetable; 2 Fruit.

Beet and Carrot Cooler

Serves: 1   *Preparation time: 5 minutes*

Ingredients
¼	cup	carrot ginger juice
¼	cup	gingered beet juice
¼	cup	coconut milk — (see *How to Make Fresh Coconut Milk* on p.135)
1	teaspoon	molasses — or to taste, with unrefined sugar or maple syrup for *vata* and *pitta*, or honey for *kapha*

A Kidney Cleanser.

Beets are cleansing and tonic laxatives with a soothing affect on the body. They promote menstruation, regulate menopause and are beneficial for anemia, the blood and liver.

Carrots are cleansing and mildly tonic vegetables. High in nutrients, anti-oxidants and anti-carcinogens, they are effective in treating acne, diarrhea, dysentery, indigestion, liver, lung and skin disorders.

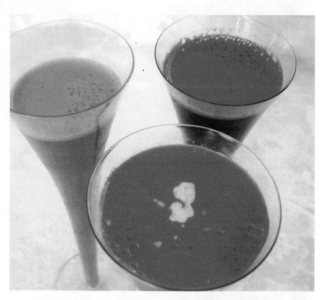

Preparation method
Mix all together.

Per Serving (excluding unknown items): 236 Calories; 15g Fat (52.8% calories from fat); 4g Protein; 26g Carbohydrate; 6g Dietary Fibre; 0mg Cholesterol; 91mg Sodium. Exchanges: 0 Grain (Starch); 3 Vegetable; 0 Fruit; 3 Fat; ½ Other Carbohydrates.

Beet, Papaya and Bean Sprout Salad

Serves: 2   **Preparation time: 10 minutes**

Ingredients
SALAD

2	cups	mung bean sprouts — 1 cup is about 2½ ounces
1	cup	papaya — ripe, medium diced, ½ cup is about 2½ ounces
½	cup	beets — peeled, small diced, ¼ cup is about 1½ ounces
4	tablespoons	currants
2	tablespoons	raw almonds, soaked overnight, skinned, rinsed and drained, chopped
2	tablespoons	parsley — chopped

DRESSING

4	tablespoons	beets — diced
4	tablespoons	coconut milk — (see *How to Make Fresh Coconut Milk* on p. 135)
¼	teaspoon	salt

Almonds are one of the best tonic foods and wonderful for rejuvenating the body. They are beneficial for asthma, chronic fatigue, coughs, low immunity and the lungs.

Bean sprouts are a Sattvic bean, great for bleeding disorders, convalescence, high blood pressure and infectious diseases.

Beets are cleansing and tonic laxatives with a soothing affect on the body. They promote menstruation, regulate menopause and are beneficial for anemia, the blood and liver.

Papaya is high in digestive enzymes, tonic and strengthening. It is beneficial for diabetes, rheumatism, hypoglycemia and parasitic infections.

Parsley is high in vitamins, minerals and anti-carcinogens. It cleanses the blood and lymph systems and is beneficial for edema, skin disorders, PMS, gall- and kidney-stones.

Preparation method
Combine salad ingredients together in a bowl. In a blender, mix puree beets and coconut milk together. Add dressing to the salad and toss well.

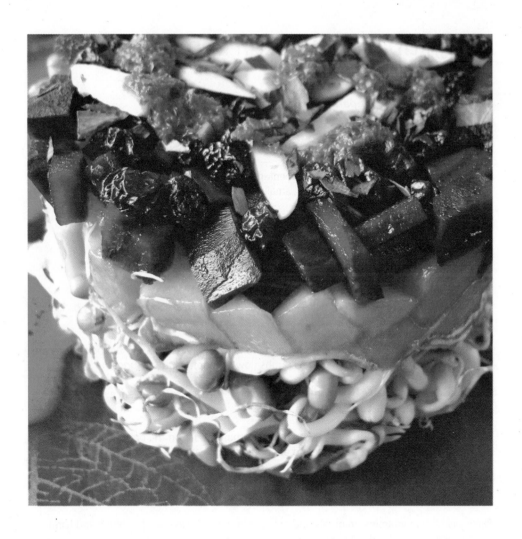

Per Serving (excluding unknown items): 255 Calories; 12g Fat (39.5% calories from fat); 8g Protein; 35g Carbohydrate; 7g Dietary Fibre; 0mg Cholesterol; 324mg Sodium. Exchanges: 0 Grain (Starch); 0 Lean Meat; 2 Vegetable; 1½ Fruit; 2½ Fat.

Carrot Ginger Juice

Serves: 1   **Preparation time: 5 minutes**

Ingredients
   8   medium   carrots
   ½   ounce   ginger — to 1 oz, or to taste

Carrots are cleansing and mildly tonic vegetables. High in nutrients, anti-oxidants and anti-carcinogens, they are effective in treating acne, diarrhea, dysentery, indigestion, liver, lung and skin disorders.

Raw ginger is added here to calm the stomach and maintain Angi (digestive enzyme functions) due to the cancer diet of mainly raw foods.

Preparation method
Place carrots and ginger in a juice extractor. Serve wtih the juice or after meals.

Per Serving (excluding unknown items): 297 Calories; 2g Fat (5.3% calories from fat); 7g Protein; 68g Carbohydrate; 19g Dietary Fibre; 0mg Cholesterol; 206mg Sodium. Exchanges: ½ Grain (Starch); 11½ Vegetable; 0 Fat.

Cider Vinaigrette

Serves: 5 tablespoons   **Preparation time: 5 minutes**

Ingredients
1	tablespoon	cider vinegar
1	teaspoon	salt
4	tablespoons	extra virgin olive oil

Preparation method
Mix cider vinegar and salt together until salt dissolves.

Add the olive oil.

Enjoy serving any raw vegetables with this dressing. Simply toss with salad ingredients. Or, with hardier raw vegetables, such as cabbage, collards, green beans and kale, you will need to massage the vegetables together with the dressing using your hands. Allow the vegetables to marinate at least 10 minutes or overnight before serving.

Note: Cider vinegar is alkaline and acceptable in a cancer diet. Olive oil is the other fat allowed in a cancer diet other than ghee.

Per Serving (excluding unknown items): 96 Calories; 11g Fat (99.3% calories from fat); 0g Protein; trace Carbohydrate; 0g Dietary Fibre; 0mg Cholesterol; 426mg Sodium. Exchanges: 2 Fat; 0 Other Carbohydrates.

Curried Avocado Carrot Soup topped with Wheatgrass Juice, Sprouts and Cilantro

Serves: 2   **Preparation time: 15 minutes**

Ingredients
Curried Avocado Carrot Soup

1	cup	carrot ginger juice
3	ounces	avocado cubes
½	teaspoon	curry powder
¼	teaspoon	salt

Wheatgrass Juice

1	cup	wheat sprouts — or wheat grass
3	tablespoons	molasses
½	cup	coconut milk — (see *How to Make Fresh Coconut Milk* on p.135)

Garnishes

¼	cup	bean sprouts
1	sprig	cilantro leaves, whole

Avocados are a tonic fruit, high in nutrients that are beneficial for the brain and blood and aid in liver, lungs, plasma and skin recuperation. They are especially good during pregnancy.

Bean sprouts are sattvic bean, great for bleeding disorders, convalescence, high blood pressure and infectious diseases.

Wheatgrass juice is strongly cleansing (therefore must be used with care) and nutritious. It cleanses the blood, reduces tumors and counters infections. Wheatgrass is used to treat arthritis, anemia, bruises, cancer, constipation, diabetes, gangrene, heavy metal toxicity, hepatitis, hypertension, hypoglycemia, obesity, prostrate, PMS and rheumatism.

Preparation method
Puree together carrot juice, avocado, curry and salt. Set aside.

Puree together wheat grass, sweetener and coconut milk. Strain and discard wheat grass. Set aside.

Spoon soup into bowls. Drizzle over wheat grass juice. Top with bean sprouts and cilantro leaves.

Per Serving (excluding unknown items): 500 Calories; 22g Fat (37.5% calories from fat); 9g Protein; 74g Carbohydrate; 11g Dietary Fibre; 0mg Cholesterol; 370mg Sodium. Exchanges: 1 1/2 Grain(Starch); 4 Vegetable; 1/2 Fruit; 4 1/2 Fat; 1 1/2 Other Carbohydrates.

Easy Curried Cream Soup

Serves: 3   **Preparation time: 5 minutes**

Ingredients

1¼	cups	coconut water — from 1 fresh coconut
¼	cup	coconut meat — from 1 fresh coconut
½	whole	avocado
½	tablespoon	curry powder
1½	tablespoons	honey — local and raw, and more for drizzling
1	teaspoon	salt

Avocados are a tonic fruit, high in nutrients that are beneficial for the brain and blood and aid in liver, lungs, plasma and skin recuperation. They are especially good during pregnancy.

Coconut is cooling, soothing and nutritious to the body. It is beneficial to the lungs and skin and helps the body recuperate from infectious diseases.

Preparation method

Puree all together.

Serve in a bowl and drizzle more honey on top.

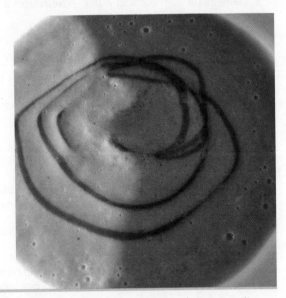

Per Serving (excluding unknown items): 132 Calories; 8g Fat (48.7% calories from fat); 2g Protein; 17g Carbohydrate; 2g Dietary Fibre; 0mg Cholesterol; 717mg Sodium. Exchanges: 0 Grain (Starch); ½ Fruit; 1½ Fat; ½ Other Carbohydrates.

Fresh Coconut Curried Salad

Serves: 1　　　　　**Preparation time: 15 minutes**

Ingredients
Raw Coconut Curry Dressing

¼	teaspoon	salt — optional
½	teaspoon	curry powder
½	whole	green chili pepper — chopped, or more to taste
1	piece	green onion — chopped
½	tablespoon	ginger — minced
1	tablespoon	raw almonds — soaked overnight, skinned, rinsed and drained, chopped
1	tablespoon	pineapple — chopped
1	tablespoon	coconut water — fresh from a green coconut
2	tablespoons	basil — chopped
¼	cup	coconut meat — fresh

Salad

½	cup	coconut meat — from a fresh green coconut, chopped
½	cup	mung bean sprouts
¼	cup	peas — freshly shucked English peas
2	tablespoons	mint — chopped
2	tablespoons	pineapples — diced
1	tablespoon	raw almonds, soaked overnight, skinned, rinsed and drained, chopped

Almonds are one of the best tonic foods and wonderful for rejuvenating the body. They are beneficial for asthma, chronic fatigue, coughs, low immunity and the lungs.

Bean sprouts are a Sattvic bean, great for bleeding disorders, convalescence, high blood pressure and infectious diseases.

Coconut is cooling, soothing and nutritious to the body. It is beneficial to the lungs and skin and helps the body recuperate from infectious diseases.

Peas reduce discharge, firm up tissues, purify blood and restore correct metabolism in the body.

Pineapple is a wonderful digestive: cleansing, diuretic, full of enzymes and they destroy intestinal worms and parasites.

Preparation method
Place all curry dressing ingredients in a food processor and puree well. Combine all salad ingredients and toss with dressing. Coconut is cooling, soothing and nutritious to the body. It is beneficial to the lungs and skin and through recuperation from infectious diseases.

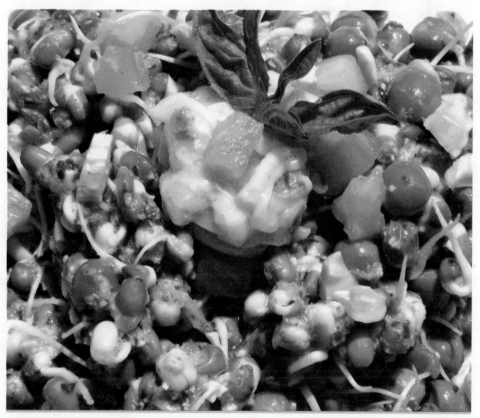

Per Serving (excluding unknown items): 433 Calories; 31g Fat (58.2% calories from fat); 12g Protein; 37g Carbohydrate; 16g Dietary Fibre; 0mg Cholesterol; 564mg Sodium. Exchanges: 1 Grain (Starch); ½ Lean Meat; 1½ Vegetable; 1 Fruit; 5½ Fat.

Fruit Shake

Serves: 3 (3 cups)   Preparation time: 5 minutes

Ingredients

1	cup	blueberries
1	cup	strawberries
4	cups	red grapes
1	teaspoon	ginger

Blueberries, grapes and strawberries all help cleanse the body of Ama.

Blueberries regulate blood sugar.

Grapes are beneficial for anemia, arthritis, gout, heart problems, hemorrhage and rheumatism.

Strawberries are beneficial for the teeth and gums, lungs and plasma.

Preparation method

Place all in blender and puree well.

Strain if desired and serve juice.

Note: Solids strained may be eaten at another time.

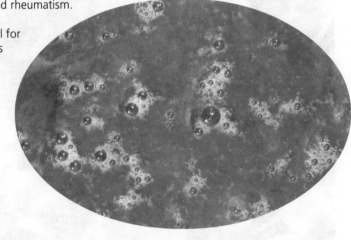

Per Serving (excluding unknown items): 124 Calories; trace Fat (2.5% calories from fat); 1g Protein; 33g Carbohydrate; 4g Dietary Fibre; 0mg Cholesterol; 6mg Sodium. Exchanges: 0 Grain (Starch); 1½ Fruit; 0 Fat.

Fruit Soup: Breakfast Porridge or Dinner Gazpacho

Serves: 2   **Preparation time: 5 minutes**

Ingredients

1½	ounces	dried apricots — about 6 pieces soaked in water overnight and drained
¼	cup	celery — chopped, about 1 oz
1	cup	cucumber — chopped, about 5 oz
1	cup	pineapple — chopped, about 5 oz
½	cup	coconut milk
½	cup	alfalfa sprouts
1	tablespoon	raw almonds, soaked overnight, skinned, rinsed and drained, chopped

Almonds are one of the best tonic foods and wonderful for rejuvenating the body. They are beneficial for asthma, chronic fatigue, coughs, low immunity and the lungs.

Alfalfa sprouts are very cooling. They are highly nutritious and cleanse the blood and lymph.

Apricots are beneficial for all lung and respiratory conditions as they cleanse and protect mucus membranes. They are a laxative and a good food for the anemic. Pregnant women can eat it in small amounts.

Celery is a Sattvic food: it cleanses the body and clears the mind. It is beneficial for reducing inflammation, urinary problems, diabetes and low blood pressure. It is an excellent food for the rejuvenation of the bones, joints, arteries and connective tissues.

Coconut is cooling, soothing and nutritious to the body. It is beneficial to the lungs and skin and helps the body recuperate from infectious diseases.

Cucumbers cool the body. As a diuretic, it is great for cleansing the system. It is beneficial for the urinary system, skin (also for burns) and reduction of inflammation. A light food, it is used to antidote heavier foods.

Pineapple is a wonderful digestive: cleansing, diuretic, full of enzymes and they destroy intestinal worms and parasites.

Preparation method

In a food processor, pulse soaked apricots and celery together until smooth. Add cucumbers, pineapples and coconut milk into the mixture and pulse to a consistency of your choice (either a rougher or smoother gazpacho).

Place in 2 bowls and garnish with alfalfa sprouts and almonds.

Per Serving (excluding unknown items): 265 Calories; 17g Fat (53.8% calories from fat); 4g Protein; 29g Carbohydrate; 5g Dietary Fibre; 0mg Cholesterol; 27mg Sodium. Exchanges: 0 Grain (Starch); 0 Lean Meat; ½ Vegetable; 1½ Fruit; 3½ Fat.

Ginger Sauce

Serves: 4 (2 to 3 cups)   Preparation time: 5 minutes

Ingredients

3	tablespoons	ginger root — minced
6	pieces	scallion — chopped
½	cup	carrot juice
1	tablespoon	olive oil
1½	teaspoons	salt

Preparation method
Puree everything
together.

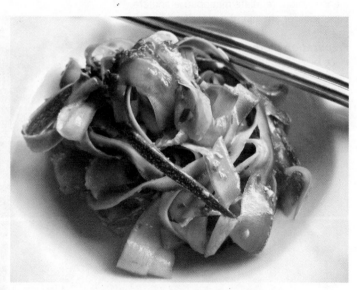

Note: A very versatile
sauce. Please look at
P.143, Sprouts Salad
with Ginger Sauce
and P.145, Vegetable
Noodles with Ginger
Sauce.

Per Serving (excluding unknown items): 52 Calories; 3g Fat (57.3% calories from fat); 1g Protein;
5g Carbohydrate; 1g Dietary Fibre; 0mg Cholesterol; 812mg Sodium. Exchanges: 1 Vegetable; ½ Fat.

Gingered Beet Juice

Serves: 2 (2 cups) **Preparation time: 5 minutes**

Ingredients
1½	pounds	beets
½	ounce	ginger

Beets are cleansing and tonic laxatives with a soothing affect on the body. They promote menstruation, regulate menopause and are beneficial for anemia, the blood and liver.

Preparation method
Place beets and ginger in a juice extractor.

Serve the juice wtih or after meals.

Raw ginger is added here to calm the stomach and maintain Angi (digestive enzyme functions) due to the cancer diet of mainly raw foods.

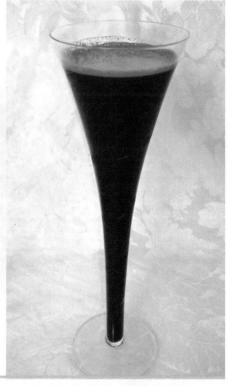

Per Serving (excluding unknown items): 245 Calories; 2g Fat (5.4% calories from fat); 9g Protein; 54g Carbohydrate; 15g Dietary Fibre; 0mg Cholesterol; 360mg Sodium. Exchanges: ½ Grain (Starch); 8½ Vegetable; 0 Fat.

Green Juice

Serves: 2   ***Preparation time: 5 minutes***

Ingredients
1	tablespoon	spirulina seaweed — powder
1	tablespoon	honey — local and raw, optional
2	cups	carrot juice — or other vegetable or fruit juice

Preparation method
Mix all together and serve.

Note: This is a 'master' spirulina juice recipe. Merely substitute any other fruit or vegetable juice for the carrot juice.

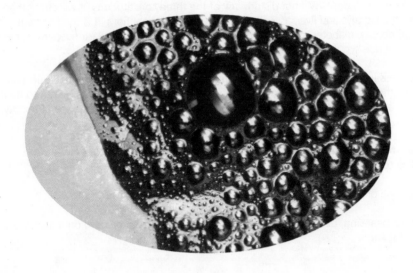

Per Serving (excluding unknown items): 129 Calories; trace Fat (2.5% calories from fat); 3g Protein; 31g Carbohydrate; 2g Dietary Fibre; 0mg Cholesterol; 76mg Sodium. Exchanges: 0 Lean Meat; 4 Vegetable; ½ Other Carbohydrates.

Green Power

Serves: 1   ***Preparation time: 5 minutes***

Ingredients
7	ounces	cucumber juice
1	ounce	wheat grass juice
1	teaspoon	ginger
1	teaspoon	spirulina powder

Cucumbers cool the body. As a diuretic, it is great for cleansing the system. It is beneficial for the urinary system, skin (also for burns) and reduction of inflammation. A light food, it is used to antidote heavier foods.

Spirulina in small doses will not disturb any of the three constitutions. It will strengthen and protect the kidneys and liver, as well as balance the intestinal flora. It is used to treat anemia, obesity, diabetes, malnourishment, hypoglycemia, arthritis, arteriosclerosis, cancer, chronic fatigue syndrome and possibly AIDS.

Wheatgrass juice is strongly cleansing (therefore must be used with care) and nutritious. It cleanses the blood, reduces tumors and counters infections. Wheatgrass is used to treat arthritis, anemia, bruises, cancer, constipation, diabetes, gangrene, heavy metal toxicity, hepatitis, hypertension, hypoglycemia, obesity, prostrate, PMS and rheumatism.

Preparation method
Blend all together.

Served wtih or after meals.

Good for cleansing, detoxifying and as a mild tonic, but not to be used on a daily basis, except for *kapha*.

Per Serving (excluding unknown items): 6 Calories; trace Fat (14.3% calories from fat); trace Protein;1g Carbohydrate; trace Dietary Fibre; 0mg Cholesterol; 1mg Sodium. Exchanges: 0 Grain (Starch); 0 Fat.

How to make Fresh Coconut Milk

Serves: 1   **Preparation time: 10 minutes**

Ingredient
1   coconut   fresh, young (like Thai green coconut)

Coconut is cooling, soothing and nutritious to the body. It is beneficial to the lungs and skin and helps the body recuperate from infectious diseases.

Preparation method
Open the coconut with a sharp cleaver.

Pour the coconut water in a blender.

Scoop out meat and place with the liquid in the blender.

Puree until smooth.

This is fresh coconut milk.

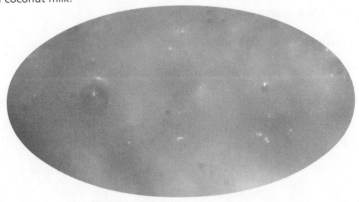

Per Serving (excluding unknown items): 1405 Calories; 133g Fat (80.2% calories from fat); 13g Protein; 60g Carbohydrate; 36g Dietary Fibre; 0mg Cholesterol; 79mg Sodium. Exchanges: 4 Fruit; 26 Fat.

How to make Mung Bean Sprouts

Serves: 4 cups   **Preparation time: 5 minutes**

Ingredient
  1   cup   mung beans — whole

Sprouting makes beans easier to digest and increases their vitamins B complex and C. When young, fresh and sprouts are around ½" long, they are highest in nutrients and cleansing.

Preparation method
Rinse mung beans.

Soak in several cups of water overnight.

The next morning, drain the water and rinse the beans. Drain well.

Place in an opaque bowl and cover with an opaque plate or cover at room temperature. Make sure that the beans are protected from the light so that they sprout.

Rinse the seeds 1 to 2 times a day.

They will be ready once they have begun to sprout, in about 2 to 3 days.

Keep rinsing 1 to 2 times a day until you use all of the sprouts.

You may remove the green hull, if you desire, by soaking the sprouts in warm water and then running water through them.

Per Serving (excluding unknown items): 718 Calories; 2g Fat (2.9% calories from fat); 49g Protein; 130g Carbohydrate; 34g Dietary Fibre; 0mg Cholesterol; 31mg Sodium. Exchanges: 8½ Grain (Starch); 3½ Lean Meat.

Minted Rose Pear Salad

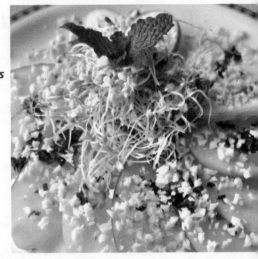

Serves: 2   **Preparation time: 5 minutes**

Ingredients

1	tablespoon	fresh mint leaves — minced
1	tablespoon	rose water
1	large	pear
½	cup	alfalfa sprouts — ½ cup is about 1 ounces
2	tablespoons	coconut meat, fresh

Coconut is cooling, soothing and nutritious to the body. It is beneficial to the lungs and skin and helps the body recuperate from infectious diseases.

Pears are cleansing especially for the liver and gall bladder, tonic for the lungs and soothing to the body. They are also a mild laxative and aid in high cholesterol, mucus and toxin build up.

Rose opens the heart and promotes positive emotions, love and compassion.

Spearmint is great for indigestion, nausea, vomiting and morning sickness.

Preparation method

Mix minced mint and rose water together. Set aside.

Slice pear nicely and fan out on 2 plates. Drizzle minted rose water on top of pear.

Place ¼ cup of sprouts at the centre of each plate and fanned out pear. Sprinkle 1 tablespoon of grated coconut over each plate. Garnish with mint leaves, if desired.

Per Serving (excluding unknown items): 70 Calories; 2g Fat (23.9% calories from fat); 1g Protein; 14g Carbohydrate; 3g Dietary Fibre; 0mg Cholesterol; 2mg Sodium. Exchanges: 0 Lean Meat; 0 Vegetable; 1 Fruit; ½ Fat.

Papaya, Grapefruit and Bean Sprout Salad

Serves: 2   **Preparation time: 10 minutes**

Ingredients
SALAD

8	ounces	papaya — sliced or diced
1	cup	mung bean sprouts
1	whole	grapefruit — segmented

DRESSING

3	tablespoons	coconut milk (see *How to Make Fresh Coconut Milk* on p.135)
1	teaspoon	molasses
1	teaspoon	ground coriander
½	teaspoon	salt — optional

GARNISH

2	tablespoons	parsley — chopped

Bean sprouts are a Sattvic bean, great for bleeding disorders, convalescence, high blood pressure and infectious diseases.

Grapefruit is a cleansing fruit, particularly if consumed in the morning. It is beneficial in the regulation of the pancreas, digestion of sugar and detoxifying from alcohol abuse.

Papaya is high in digestive enzymes, tonic and strengthening. It is beneficial for diabetes, rheumatism, hypoglycemia and parasitic infections.

Preparation method
Combine papaya, sprouts and grapefruit together.

Mix dressing ingredients together and toss with salad ingredients.

Garnish with parsley.

Per Serving (excluding unknown items): 170 Calories; 8g Fat (39.6% calories from fat); 4g Protein; 25g Carbohydrate; 4g Dietary Fibre; 0mg Cholesterol; 543mg Sodium. Exchanges: 0 Grain(Starch); ½ Vegetable; 1 Fruit; 1½ Fat; 0 Other Carbohydrates.

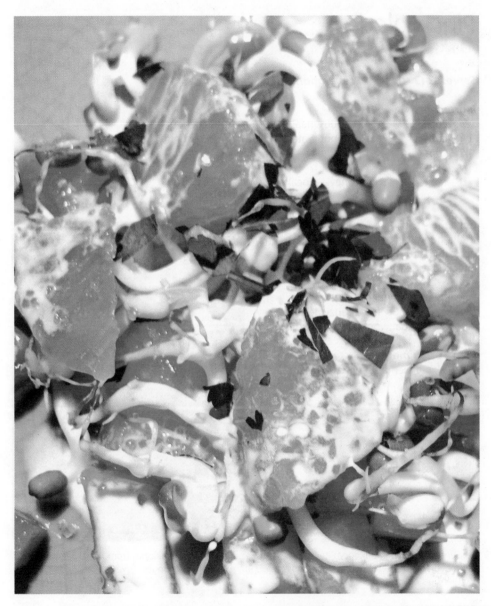

Pina Colada

Serves: 3 (3 cups)   **Preparation time: 5 minutes**

Ingredients

¼	cup	coconut meat — from 1 fresh coconut
1¼	cups	coconut water — from 1 fresh coconut
1½	cups	pineapple — fresh, chopped
1½	cups	water
3	tablespoons	honey — local and raw
3	sprigs	mint

Coconut is cooling, soothing and nutritious to the body. It is beneficial to the lungs and skin and helps the body recuperate from infectious diseases.

Pineapple is a wonderful digestive: cleansing, diuretic, full of enzymes and they destroy intestinal worms and parasites.

Preparation method

Place all in a blender and puree until smooth.

Serve.

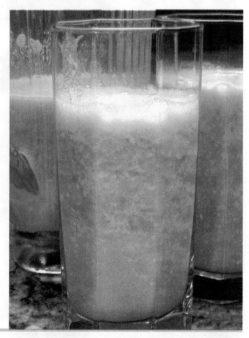

Per Serving (excluding unknown items): 147 Calories; 3g Fat (15.8% calories from fat); 1g Protein; 32g Carbohydrate; 2g Dietary Fibre; 0mg Cholesterol; 9mg Sodium. Exchanges: 0 Vegetable; 1 Fruit; ½ Fat; 1 Other Carbohydrates.

Sprout Power Wrap

Serves: 4   **Preparation time: 10 minutes**

Ingredients
Mung Sprout Avocado Spread

1	cup	mung bean sprouts
1	small	avocado — around 4 ounces of avocado meat
1	clove	garlic — chopped
¼	whole	green chili pepper — chopped
1	tablespoon	water — add more for a more fluid consistency
½	teaspoon	salt
¼	teaspoon	black pepper

For the Wraps

12	pieces	lettuce leaves — any hard stems removed
2	ounces	sprouts — your choice of alfalfa, clover or other

(Sliced raw vegetables can be included in the wraps as well, such as: thinly sliced peppers, cucumbers, scallions, carrots and beets.)

Alfalfa sprouts are very cooling. They are highly nutritious and cleanse the blood and lymph.

Avocados are a tonic fruit, high in nutrients that are beneficial for the brain and blood and aid in liver, lungs, plasma and skin recuperation. They are especially good during pregnancy.

Bean sprouts are a Sattvic bean, great for bleeding disorders, convalescence, high blood pressure and infectious diseases.

Lettuce is a cooling cleanser that calms the nerves. It is beneficial for urinary inflammations, obesity and plasma purification.

Preparation method
Place mung bean sprouts, avocado, garlic, lemon juice and salt in a processor and puree until smooth. Set aside.

Wash and dry lettuce leaves well. Place some spread on lettuce leaves and top with some sprouts. You may add other vegetables for colour and taste, as desired. Roll lettuce leaves and serve.

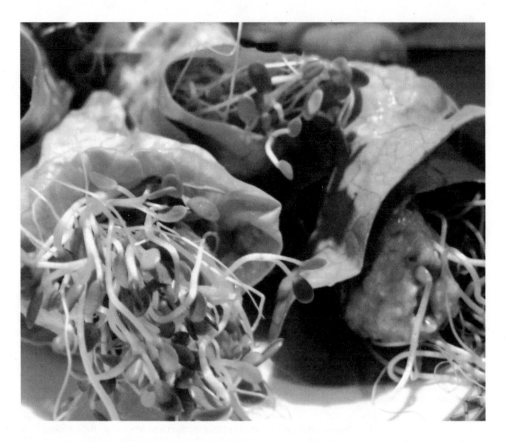

Serving idea: You can use this mung sprout avocado spread as a dip or spread or dressing for a salad or sauce for vegetable noodles (please see *Vegetable Noodles with Ginger Sauce* on p. 145).

Per Serving (excluding unknown items): 98 Calories; 8g Fat (64.9% calories from fat); 3g Protein; 7g Carbohydrate; 2g Dietary Fibre; 0mg Cholesterol; 277mg Sodium. Exchanges: 0 Grain(Starch); ½ Vegetable; 0 Fruit; 1½ Fat.

Sprouts Salad with Ginger Sauce

Serves: 1   **Preparation time: 5 minutes**

Ingredients
½	whole	avocado
½	cup	tomatoes
1	cup	sprouts
3	tablespoons	ginger sauce

Preparation method
Place ingredients on a plate.

Drizzle sauce on top.

Serve and enjoy!

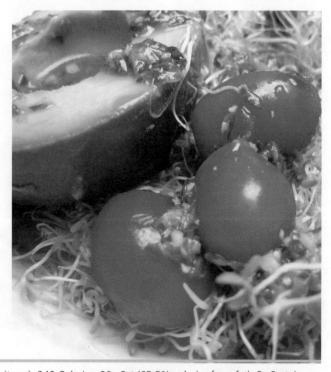

Per Serving (excluding unknown items): 249 Calories; 20g Fat (65.5% calories from fat); 5g Protein; 19g Carbohydrate; 5g Dietary Fibre; 0mg Cholesterol; 934mg Sodium. Exchanges: 2 Vegetable; ½ Fruit; 4 Fat.

Sweet Fruit Lassi

Serves: 3   **Preparation time: 5 minutes**

Ingredients

¼	cup	coconut meat — from 1 coconut
1¼	cups	coconut water — from 1 coconut
1½	cups	papaya
1½	cups	water
3½	tablespoons	honey — local and raw
¾	teaspoon	cardamom

Preparation method

Puree all together.

Serve.

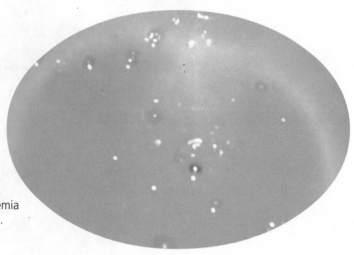

Note: As mangoes are potentially acidic forming, papaya is substituted here in the lassi. Papaya is high in digestive enzymes, tonic and strengthening. It is beneficial for diabetes, rheumatism, hypoglycemia and parasitic infections.

Per Serving (excluding unknown items): 173 Calories; 3g Fat (12.9% calories from fat); 1g Protein; 39g Carbohydrate; 3g Dietary Fibre; 0mg Cholesterol; 9mg Sodium. Exchanges: 0 Grain (Starch); 1 Fruit; ½ Fat; 1½ Other Carbohydrates.

Vegetable Noodles with Ginger Sauce

Serves: 1   **Preparation time: 5 minutes**

Ingredients
1	piece	zucchini or other vegetable noodle (look at serving idea notes)
3	tablespoons	ginger sauce
1	teaspoon	cilantro leaves, whole — minced

Preparation method
Use a peeler to make vegetable noodles. Mix with ginger sauce. Top with cilantro and serve.

Serving idea: Vegetable 'noodles' can be any vegetable that can be grated or shredded or sliced thinly with a peeler to create 'noodles', such as carrots, beets, squash, zucchini, cabbage. Garnishes can also include other chopped vegetables to resemble a stir-fry, such as peppers, celery, mushrooms, peas, etc.

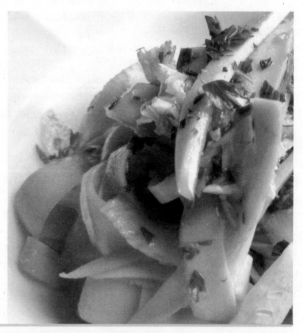

Per Serving (excluding unknown items): 86 Calories; 4g Fat (39.3% calories from fat); 3g Protein; 11g Carbohydrate; 3g Dietary Fibre; 0mg Cholesterol; 920mg Sodium. Exchanges: 2 Vegetable; 1 Fat.

REFERENCE

1. M. Napier, Kristine. *Eat to Heal*. Clayton: Warner Books. 1998.

2. Wigmore, Ann. *Be Your Own Doctor*. New York: Avery Publisher Group. 2nd Edition. 1983.

3. Sharon, Michael. *Nutrients A to Z*. London: Prion Books. 2004.

4. Aman. *Medicinal Secrets of Your Food*. Health Research. 1979

5. Ritcliff, J.D. *I am Joe's Body*. New York: Berkley Publishing Group. 1982.

6. E. Larson, David. *Mayo Clinic Family Health Book*. New York: William Morrow & Company. 1990.

7. Hilgard, Ernest R., L. Atkinson, Rita, and C. Atkinson, Richard. *Introduction to Psychology*. Harcourt Brace Jovanorich Inc. 1979.

8. R. Clark, Hulda. *The Cure for All Cancers*. New Century Press. 1993.

9. A. Baron, Robert. *Psychology*. Prentice Hall College Division. 4th Edition. 1999.

10. Silva, Jose and Miele, Philip. *The Silva Mind Control Method*. Pocket Books. 1991.

11. Silva, Jose with B. Stone, Robert. *The Silva Mind Control Method For Getting Help From Your Other Side*. Pocket Books. 1989.

12. Sivananda, Swami. *Health and Hygiene*. Divine Life Society. 6th Edition. 1996.

13. Sivananda, Swami. Japa Yoga, Divine Life Society. 11th Edition 1994.

14. Sivananda, Swami. *Mind – Its Mysteries and Control*. Divine Life Society. 12th Edition. 1994.

15. Sivananda, Swami. *Sure Ways for Success in Life & God Realization*. Divine Life Society. 13th Edition. 1990.

16. Sivananda, Swami. *Concentration and Meditation*. Divine Life Society. 8th Edition. 1990.

17. Ramacharaka,Yogi. *Hatha Yoga*. Montana, USA: Kessinger Publishing. 1998.

18. Ramacharaka,Yogi. *Fourteen Lessons in Yogi Philosophy and Oriental Occultism*. Montana, USA: Kessinger Publishing. 2003.

19. Yogananda, Paramahamsa. *Autobiography of a Yogi*. Los Angeles, CA: Self Realisation Fellowship Publisher. 1979.

20. *Hatha Yoga Pradipika*. Munger: Bihar School of Yoga. 1985.

21. Satyananda Saraswati, Swami. *Asana Pranayama Mudra Bandha*. Munger: Bihar School of Yoga. 2nd Edition. 1971.

22. Satyananda Saraswati, Swami. *Yoga Nidra*. Munger: Bihar School of Yoga.

23. Satyananda Saraswati, Swami. *Meditation from Tantra*. 5th Edition. 1983.

24. Satyananda Saraswati, Swami. *Self Realisation*. Munger: Bihar School of Yoga.

25. Satyananda Saraswati, Swami. *Yogic Cure for Common Diseases*. Munger: Bihar School of Yoga. 1983.

26. *Teaching of Swami Satyananda Saraswati*. Munger: Bihar School of Yoga. Vol. I. First Australian Edition. 1981, Vol. IV. 4th Enlarged Edition. 1986. Vol. V. 1986.

27. Devananda, Visnu. *Meditation and Mantras*. New Delhi: Motilal Banarsidass. 1999.

28. Kok Sui, Choa. *The Ancient Science & Art of Pranic Healing*. Institute for Inner Studies. 1987.

29. Muktananda Saraswati, Swami. *Nawayogini Tantra*. 1975.

30. Satyananda Saraswati, Swami. *Yoga Education for Children*. 1985.

INDEX

Recipe Index